ATOMIC
GOLF

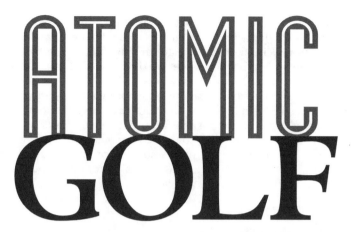

ATOMIC GOLF

*The Alternative to Swing Gurus,
Pie-in-the-Sky Theories, Perfect Greens,
and Everything Else That's Failed*

STEVE MICHALIK
MR. USA • MR. AMERICA • MR. UNIVERSE

& MICHAEL MANAVIAN
PROFESSIONAL GOLF COACH

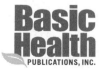

Basic
Health
PUBLICATIONS, INC.

The information contained in this book is based upon the research and personal and professional experiences of the author. It is not intended as a substitute for consulting with your physician or other healthcare provider. Any attempt to diagnose and treat an illness should be done under the direction of a healthcare professional.

The publisher does not advocate the use of any particular healthcare protocol but believes the information in this book should be available to the public. The publisher and author are not responsible for any adverse effects or consequences resulting from the use of the suggestions, preparations, or procedures discussed in this book. Should the reader have any questions concerning the appropriateness of any procedures or preparation mentioned, the author and the publisher strongly suggest consulting a professional healthcare advisor.

Basic Health Publications, Inc.
28812 Top of the World Drive
Laguna Beach, CA 92651
949-715-7327 • www.basichealthpub.com

Library of Congress Cataloging-in-Publication Data
Michalik, Steve.
   The alternative to swing gurus, pie-in-the-sky theories, perfect greens, and everything else that's failed / Steve Michalik and Michael Manavian.
      p. cm.
   Includes bibliographical references and index.
   ISBN 978-1-59120-188-5
   1. Swing (Golf) 2. Golf—Training. 3. Physical fitness.
I. Manavian, Michael. II. Title.

   GV979.S9M5133   2008
   796.352'3—dc22

                                          2008026121

Editor: Cheryl Hirsch
Photographers: Larry Tallis (exercise photos) and Denny (vintage photos)
Design/Typesetting: Gary A. Rosenberg • Photo layout: Theresa Wiscovitch
Cover design: Mike Stromberg

Printed in the United States of America

10   9   8   7   6   5   4   3   2   1

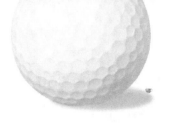

Contents

Part Three • The Atomic Golfer

Dedicated to . . .

We, the authors, would like to dedicate this book to all of the suffering golfers who have gone through life playing this game so poorly; to those dedicated souls who have yearned for the truth and have now all but given up hope; to those who have sought out countless hours of golf instruction that yielded no results; to the professional golf instructor whose passion is to give back to the game by improving another's ability; and to the beginning golfer who has made the decision to pick up this game with the vigor and zest that we all experienced long ago.

To all of you, may this book fulfill your quest for playing this precise and rewarding game at its highest level.

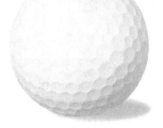

Preface

The golfer: who is this person? What would possess someone to take up such an impossible sport? Is he or she a competitive athlete? A sadist? A person who's just crazy about the game? The golfer spends long hours visualizing that perfect shot. They dream of making that impossible putt, being under par, and raising the trophy at dusk on the eighteenth green. This would be a lot easier to accomplish if they knew some fundamental truths about not only the physical side, but also the psychological side, of playing golf. What is this truth, you ask? *Webster's Dictionary* (10th ed., 1995) says, "It is a state in accordance with fact or reality, experience, accurate, right and correct." In writing this book, we strip away false data and replace it with truth.

With that said, the accounts of the authors shared here are what we saw and experienced to be the truth. Let the record and responsibility of the context of this text stand.

Millions upon millions of words have been written about every facet and aspect of golf. They cover all bases and viewpoints, both physiological and psychological. It is our belief that less than 5 percent of this information comes close to bearing any workable knowledge that you can actually use and apply to golf. Therefore, the bulk of this book is devoted to bringing forth a full understanding of the game and correcting that which is misunderstood. Welcome to the journey. We can assure you it's a fascinating one. Our mission is simple: to bring forth the basic information needed to produce a better golfer.

People have asked us, why write this book? With its different approach to the physiology and psychology involved in the game of golf, it is certain to stir up controversy. Our response is simple: it is worth anything that we may encounter to reveal the truth. As in all the books we write.

After decades of observation, data collection, and application, we felt it was time to present our findings to the world. This technology, this data, this truth, should not be lost. Confusion and controversy should be put to rest. This data need not be boring or complicated. It should be rapidly assimilated and applied. True understanding of the information should expose the mountain of false information associated with the game of golf and help millions of misguided golfers. The noble sport of golf, steeped as it is in tradition and history, deserves this different approach.

So, to those who would disgrace this majestic field of endeavor with false hope, malice, ignorance, and misinformation, let them be exposed for who and what they are. We put forth that a life based on truth will always, in the end, surpass a life based on a lie. We will attack in the name of this truth and release those prisoners burdened by frustration and failure. And, in conclusion, we wish to thank all those past and present who worked without notoriety or reward so that others may not play this gallant sport in vain.

Introduction

*I*n life, there are certain disciplines that govern each and every intention we undertake. If you apply these disciplines to anything in life, you will succeed. This brings us to the game of golf, where the mind and body must mesh in a symphony of action.

Practice, persistence, and purpose will get you skill, but to constantly deliver that skill is another thing entirely. A strong body and mind are like a well-oiled machine—powerful, stable, and enduring—and necessary if you are to deliver your skill consistently and become the Atomic Golfer. As used in this book, the word "atomic" means indivisible. An atomic operation, or atomicity, implies an operation that must be performed entirely or not at all.

Up until now, the golf world had not made this mind/body connection. After all, look at the physiques of golfers. Most are fat, beer-bellied, middle-aged men who smoke cigars. They are not going to grace the cover of *Muscle and Fitness* magazine anytime soon. Articles are constantly written about how golfers are not athletes, and they're right! For those who have just recently caught the fitness craze (a reaction called "the Tiger Woods effect"), their exercise regimens consist mainly of stretching, which does little to improve their game and mental focus.

In this book, we teach you what skills are necessary to play and win at golf. But we go two steps further: we show you 1) how to build a better machine, which will make you stronger and faster and produce so much torque that the ball will explode off your club, and 2) how to build an equally strong mind, which will allow that to happen. We will be revealing the trappings of the mind and explaining how they play a part in your success and failure on the golf course.

Some people believe that intelligence is a substitute for experience; others feel that experience is senior to intelligence. Truth of the matter is, there must be a balance of both. This will allow you to apply the correct amount of force at the precise time, in the exact direction, in order to project the ball where you want it to go.

THE CHALLENGES—AND GIFTS—OF GOLF

The game of golf has been around for roughly 500 years, and yet the tiny idiosyncrasies that have made this a difficult game continue to frustrate nearly everyone who plays it.

Golf transcends other games by its mere design. It requires the assembly of a golf swing that couples gracefulness with power, and yet asks you to combine that with a deft sense of touch. It physically demands the highest levels of performance for well over four hours for four days of seventy-two-hole championship play, in conditions that are aerobically demanding and in environments that can range from desert heat to winter's frigid chill.

At the same time, it creates the ultimate test. This test mentally challenges the seeker to attain perfection, while bombarding its participants with the fiercest distractions and at the same time tempting players to beat the game. Now this is a game! A balanced game, one that equally tests the mind's focus, the body's rudiments, and the player's technique.

Golf offers no guarantee for success, no multimillion dollar compensation packages for injuries or bench time. What's required is to show up and shoot your best. You're in complete control, allowing for 100 percent responsibility based on your outcome. There is no opponent knocking your ball away, or hip-checking you as you attempt a shot. You start equally with those you battle, and through your creation is your fate determined.

Golf is a game of integrity, honor, and tradition, the rules of which are self-imposed and self-enforced. It is a game whose records have not faded, but rather have stood the test of time in an ever-advancing, technology-driven industry.

Few other sports present its participants an opportunity for such grandeur as golf. Golf provides a camaraderie that creates enduring friendships. It offers the passion that arises with skilled execution. It does not discriminate or hold bias against one's background, size, or age. It is encompassed by vast landscapes set in nature's most astonishing creations while bestowing upon the participant the capacity to provide a lifetime full of enjoyment. Ah yes, golf is truly a game of honor. It instills in us a personal dignity, a strength of character, and ethics.

A NEW STANDARD *AND* A NEW APPROACH

The original objective of golf still remains quite simple: to put the ball in the hole with the least amount of strokes. Since the inception of the game, the solutions to achieve this task have eluded all those who have played it. Society's most established masterminds have collided with the task, reaching conclusions that seem to provide further diluted data and invoke more unwarranted confusion.

For the most part, the search to bring about a better golf game for the masses has always been the intention of researchers. The dilemma they faced was never in the search, but rather, it was in the "solutions" that they provided, which never produced a champion or recurring champions. The best instructors of every era have yet to create players who can win and produce championships consistently. One-hit wonders and a variety of "could-have-beens" fill their stables in the hope that if a few players win a few events over the course of a lifetime, then the instructor is regarded as a guru who can somehow magically open the gates to the secrets of golfing Valhalla—which, unfortunately, they've proven they still cannot do.

The meek standards that have been used to measure greatness are coming to an end. Those who venture to accept another student will create the same result in every student they gather under their wings. The creation of champions, who can produce championships with increasingly better results day in and day out, is now the new standard. To duplicate this with uniformity is truly our goal. And that is all that can be asked.

HOW TO USE THIS BOOK

This book is compiled so that you, the reader, will gain maximum results. Part One, The Atomic Mind, uncovers what it is that holds you back mentally and the procedures you can do to gain that mental edge. Part Two, The Atomic Body, shows how you can prepare your body to respond with power to your command without qualification. And, in Part Three, The Atomic Golfer, you will discover technically exactly what it is you need to do, how to do it, and what is in the way that prevented you from doing it in the past.

What we have amassed here is the truth, with no stone left unturned. Our focus here will point out why you haven't been able to play your best so that now you can. You will identify the problem that is troubling you most and attack it from all angles with workable solutions.

The steps to fix your body's rudiments are here.

The processes to laser your mind's focus and sharpness are here.

The mysteries of a powerful golf swing with control and accuracy are revealed here.

Read and apply what is written here 100 percent and you will never be the same golfer, nor the same person, again.

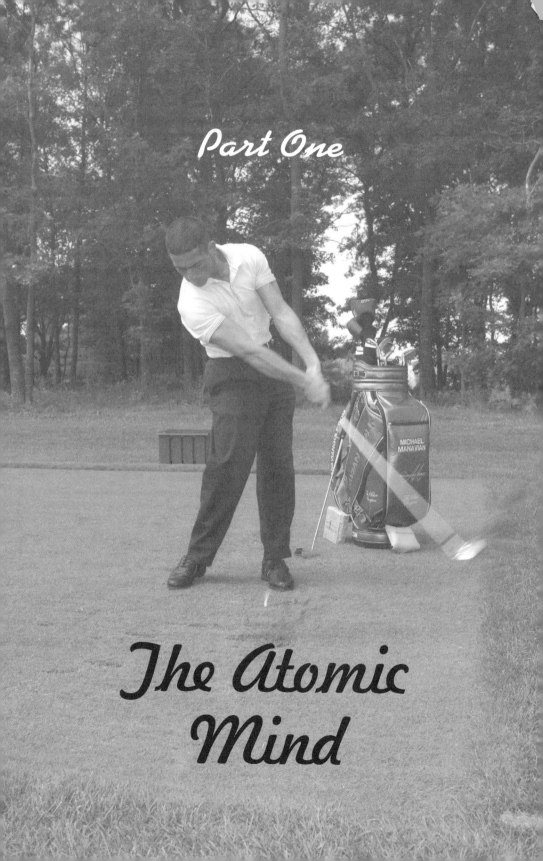

Part One

The Atomic
Mind

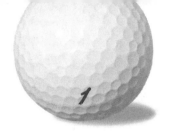

The Ultimate Goal

*T*o fully understand any activity, goal, or purpose—be it golf, climbing Mt. Everest, or even going into work on a daily basis—one must look at the "self," the force behind these objectives. The "basic basic" of all things, the ultimate beginning from which all things spring, is still you. To truly play any sport is basically to challenge the universe. To win we must know the knowable, so let's try.

THE PLAYING FIELD

We live in a playing field called the universe. In the playing field there are space, time, objects, energy, and life force (more about these later). The objective of this game is simple: to survive. From our unknown beginnings to our ultimate and infinite destination, the single purpose of every human being is to *be*. This doesn't mean you will. What it does mean is that you are driven to carry on for as long as possible. We suppose that if dinosaurs could have, they would have chosen to never perish. The dominant life forms change, but the life force itself is infinite. A human being's mind is their ultimate survival weapon. The brain is the weapon of choice for our species. Isn't it interesting that this same mechanism will ultimately be what destroys us?

Simply being, therefore, is the ultimate dynamic of life. To avoid pain and unhappiness and to strive toward pleasure and happiness is our reward. To alter from this brings different degrees of unhappiness. The more unhappiness, the greater the state of nonsurvival and the further away we are from surviving and achieving our goals.

There are different degrees of survival that permeate our lives from hour to hour and day to day due to the forces and flux of the universe, which we have no control over. What we do have control over is how we deal with this flux.

MASTERING LIFE

This playing field—your life—is replete with barriers and rewards. These positive and negative forces affect us physically and mentally by raising us up and then casting us down. These variables of happiness, pain, and unhappiness are not arbitrary. A calm mind and a silent being can rise above most any negative force and will keep climbing toward the ultimate state of *being* self. The more you know (not memorization-acquired knowledge) and learn how to know, the more you move away from aberration and the closer you get to self-determinism. As your powers of perception increase, as the ability to perceive things as they actually are (not as you have been taught, not what you have been made to believe), the less robotic you will act. As your powers of perception decrease, the less sentient you become and the closer you get to the intelligence of an animal. Only through the force and power of the mind can you move toward this fundamental state.

This path of selfhood travels a dual road: there is pain, which leads to destruction or nonsurvival, and there is pleasure, which leads to production or survival. People will put up with a lot of pain to experience a little pleasure. To obtain happiness, it is necessary to be successful at surviving. The more knowledge and intelligence you possess, the greater your ability to perceive and resolve problems. This ultimately leads to pleasure and immortality—if you can master this, mastering golf will seem simple.

The Inner Workings of the Mind

*B*efore you can understand the Atomic Golf System, you must first understand that you are not your mind and you are not your body. You are simply you—a being. You occupy a body that uses a brain as a computer and its software—the mind. This mind determines your future successes and failures. Even a little understanding of how the mind works will put you at a great advantage over others, for little to nothing is taught about the mind, and less is understood about it.

What do we know about the human mind? The mind can be considered as the sum of three parts, as we know it today:

- The computing mind acts like a computer; it is responsible for computing data, gathering and analyzing information.

- The stimulus/response mind functions as a conduit, relaying information between the internal environment within the body and the external environment outside it; this part of the mind cannot reason, it reacts.

- The body-mind regulates all bodily functions, such as DNA replication, breathing, heart rate, body temperature, digestion, sleep, and other physiological functions.

THE COMPUTING MIND

The computing mind is the most recently evolved part of the mind. It is considered the general—the leader—and is responsible for resolving problems relative to living. It organizes responses to complex problems, plans steps to an objective, searches memory for relevant experience, and guides behavior with verbal skills and socially appropriate ways of responding. The computing mind is incapable of making a mistake. It is a perfect machine. If given perfect data, perfect conclusions will arise. This mind is infallible.

However, the mind's computer is only as good as the data with which it operates. The problem arises, then, with the data presented to it. False conclusions and distorted solutions will result when the offered data is inaccurate. This data, whether it is real or unreal, correct or incorrect, is stored in the memory. As it is taken in from the senses, it is filed in separate areas within the memory. For this mind, perception is reality. The computing mind can instantly cross-reference these memory areas to come up with a concept, decision, or conclusion. If the data is correct, a correct conclusion will result. However, the computing mind cannot determine if any or all of the data it is given is aberrant. It can merely formulate a solution based on the data it is given. Everything conceptualized is stored in the memory forever. (Now you should begin to realize that if you're not in a healthy mental shape, your golf game becomes one of pure randomness, full of maybes, hopes, and false conclusions.)

The computing mind works hard to keep the body running soundly, performing endless tasks in everyday life. It can develop certain working patterns it feels will aid in its survival (toward pleasure). An endless number of learned patterns can be stored to memory, such as tasks like eating, walking, playing a sport, talking, riding a bike, and so forth. And here is the sportsman's dilemma! Once you have learned how to swing a golf club correctly, why should it be so difficult to duplicate the motion every time? The golf swing is stored in the computing mind's memory and becomes a learned pattern. What is stopping you from performing that swing perfectly forever? This involves further investigation. Read on, and we will unravel this mystery.

THE STIMULUS/RESPONSE MIND

The stimulus/response mind does not think or reason; it simply reacts to the environment, without contemplating the consequences of its actions, in an endless struggle to protect you and keep you alive. It is a slave to mis-emotion (any unpleasant emotion such as antagonism, grief, fear) and mis-thought (any thought that doesn't line up with reality). Before the development of the computing mind, our ancestors relied on this mind for survival. While the stimulus/response mind may have kept our early ancestors alive, through time and evolution, it became less of an asset as people began using the analytical part of their minds for survival. Like most other useless functions, the stimulus/response mind should have become extinct, but it didn't and the joke's on us.

So how does this stimulus/response mind act on you? It happens when the computing mind goes off-line—that's how! The stimulus/response mind is then free to take over and run you as if you were once again a caveman. Unfortunately for us, this mind does not think or analyze. It sees everything as being equal to everything else, and it is unable to differentiate.

What causes the computing mind to go off-line, you may wonder? It can happen in moments of physical, mental, or emotional overload—moments when you are experiencing massive confusion or doubt, intense physical pain, or emotional trauma such as loss and disappointment. It can also happen when you're out of present time due to drugs, alcohol, anesthesia, or even daydreaming. When your mind is off-line, you're not fully there, and you can't concentrate or fully observe what you perceive. In short, you are mentally absent. The stimulus/response mind will then kick in, instantly taking control over the job of the computing mind and will run the body. During these times, the stimulus/response mind runs the body on automatic. It records everything it senses and stores the data to memory.

The problem is that the stimulus/response mind records everything whether it's real or unreal, correct or incorrect, rational or irrational, and deposits the data as fact alongside the data entered in the computing mind. When the computing mind comes back online and brings you back to the present, it doesn't know of this stimulus/response mind's misdeeds and uses the new data along with its own to handle problems and find solutions. This explains the confusion on the golf course of why you "can" one day and you "can't" the next. You think you're swinging the golf club correctly but, in actuality, your body is being driven by false data and misemotions.

The source of all aberrations (distortion), problems, or the inability on the golf course to repeat success can be traced back to the stimulus/response mind's deposits of incorrect data and solutions in your computing mind's memory. The mind is recording all the time, 24/7, whether you're awake or asleep. These recordings are made by either the analytical/computing mind or the stimulus/response mind, and they remain in the memory forever. Since these recordings contain information drafted from the senses, emotions, pain, and all conclusions, whether right or wrong, it is important to remain in present time so you can use the computing mind to perceive reality for what it is, and so that correct decisions can be made when you're getting ready to hit a shot. If incorrect data is stored next to correct data due to this lapse by the computing mind, then subsequent solutions, though based on false information, will appear correct. Remember, the analyzer is infallible. It will give answers based on what it has stored in memory. In your viewpoint, you are doing everything perfect, but the stimulus/response mind feels it has the answers to your golf swing. In other words, who is really playing golf? Is it you? Or all the false data acting as you? The computing mind does not store painful incidents or events, either physical or emotional. These are recorded by the stimulus/response mind and sent to memory. This is the reason for all errors in judgment and aberrant solutions, including slicing, hooking, distance control, misreading putts, and so forth. It is this restimulation, or reenactment, in the environment that prevents you from having your best game.

Restimulations

A restimulation happens like this: when anything in the environment duplicates what your senses recorded through the stimulus/response mind (failure, pain, loss, mis-emotion, etc.), you will experience the same feeling, sensation, pain, or emotion, all over again, as if the original experience just happened. Any analytical decision at that moment would be impossible, for all conclusions would be based upon information coming from the memory of the stimulus/response recording: good, bad, or anything in between. At these times, it is best to keep your thoughts and focus steady. (More on these mental techniques in Chapter 6.) You cannot take life into the game of golf.

Let's look at a simple example of the power one of these old memories can have. A young girl is at home in her bedroom. It is night, and she is sleeping. She is awakened by thunder and is frightened. She leaves her room to find her parents. She's in the dark, and the smell of cookies her mother recently baked is still in the air. The house is cool. She stumbles in the hallway and hits her head. For a moment, her computing mind shuts down. Instead, her stimulus/response mind records everything—the thunder, the darkness, the cool air, the smell of cookies, the head bump, and so on. It records this data in no particular order. Now, years later, the same girl is walking by a bakery and smells fresh baked cookies. She suddenly feels kind of frightened, her head begins to hurt slightly, and she can't figure out why. This girl, now a woman, is somewhere and hears thunder. She feels frightened, a little chill comes over her, and she can't understand why she's afraid. It's the old memory that is being restimulated in the present. These episodes may come in any order and in any magnitude. When this happens, it takes you out of the moment and puts you in a sort of half here/half there state. You can't demonstrate skill if you're half here.

As you can see, a memory filled with this stuff can interfere with the decision-making process, causing wrong actions, unfounded fears, phobias, and anxieties. Every time you feel uncomfortable around someone or in some place, or experience sudden pains in the body for no apparent reason—if you make the same mistakes repeatedly—if things are going great and then, for no apparent reason, they take a turn for the worse—it's due to a restimulation of events stored in the memory. You'll never play golf to your full potential in this state.

This stimulus/response mind demands sympathy as a solution. Feelings of need and dependency on others for survival, insecurities, and low self-esteem are all unnatural. They are, however, powerful components of the stimulus/response mind and will cause pain, illness, and even death if not obeyed. This mind demands that it must be—*dead right!*

THE BODY-MIND

Where exactly is this stimulus/response mind located? One can only speculate, but with good reason, some evidence, and perhaps a little history of the organism, we can draw some conclusions.

All life began from one-celled organisms. This single cell must have had a mind in order to follow DNA's orders. This one cell divided into many to become an organization of cells, and eventually it formed into an organ. The organs joined other organs in a structure, which over time evolved into a human being. This structure, comprised of cells, forms the living tissue of the body, from bone to brain, all functioning together through collective thinking. Like a beehive, they all work for the collective—the body. This is your body-mind.

As previously explained, as our ancestors evolved they developed a computing mind that was capable of analytical thinking and reasoning and that was used to further ensure survival. The stimulus/response mind would take over to ensure the survival of the organism when the analytical mind was compromised. This stimulus/response mind is a collective of all the cells of the body and acts as a unit and becomes a cellular commander. If, for any reason, the cellular commander feels the computing mind cannot fulfill the job of survival, it will take over until the danger passes and the computing mind is able to regain control.

It is our strong belief that your DNA is a storage area for all the action, incidents, and events that have ever happened in your ancestral line. Everything your parents did, their parents did, and so forth has been recorded and stored as data. All your urges, phobias, fears, and other mis-emotions and destructive thoughts are forever present in your DNA and influence all the cells of your body. All disease, sickness, and strengths and weaknesses are stored in your DNA. You are basically a prisoner of your ancestry. Your DNA works in tandem with the stimulus/response mind by being a library of information—bad or good—that can be called upon to solve problems.

Unfortunately, this body-mind stimulus/response mind records data from the environment without analyzing it or interpreting it. What comes in, comes in, and it is literally interpreted. For example, a man walks across an unpaved road and stumbles. He falls, hurts himself, and blacks out for a moment. The computing mind shuts down. The body-mind takes over, and the stimulus/response mind takes over, recording everything literally. A person walking by, sees the man, and comments loud enough for him to hear, "That spot in the road can be a real pain in the neck." This is recorded literally in the mind of the fallen man. In the future, anything that resembles a spot in the road, whether it's a painted spot or broken pavement that looks like a spot, has the potential to evoke a "pain in the neck" for our poor victim. The stimulus/response mind has drawn a conclusion that survival of this organism requires bringing on neck pain any time he sees a spot in the road.

Now, just think about the possibilities when you're under anesthesia at the dentist's office, or having some operation, and a doctor or a nurse makes a comment—any comment, from the procedure to what they're having for dinner—your stimulus/response mind records it all. You get the full dose! From that moment on, any time a similar scenario takes place, whether in real life or in a movie, whatever you recorded will affect you to some degree, and you will not know why. There will be hidden commands, suggestion, phobias, body pains, sickness, allergies, accidents, and so forth. Anything that was said could be literally interpreted by the mind as a survival trait. When the restimulation takes place, the ability to reason shuts down. The ability to know or learn shuts down. Your ability to differentiate is impaired, and you think only in terms of identification or association of something to something else. There are no facts, only scrambled data.

Here's another example. Let's say our guy on the pavement suffers extreme emotional pain and humiliation. The computing mind will also shut down due to emotional pain. A woman comes along and comforts him. She may have a particular look about her, or smell of a particular fragrance. The stimulus/response mind will record all this as pleasurable and pro-survival. Now, every time this guy sees a woman who looks, smells, or wears similar clothing to the one who provided comfort, he will feel good and be drawn to her. He may even eventually choose to marry based on these qualities. He will not know why; he will think he's in love. He will believe he has met his soul mate when, in fact, all he's encountered is his stimulus/response mind.

SO, WHO'S IN CONTROL?

Have you ever been in a situation where you just can't seem to think straight, or you can't figure out how to make that next drive or putt? This happens when your conscious, computing mind is shut down or only partially working. The individual on the course is not you; they are a restimulation of someone who was recorded during a time of pain—physical or emotional—while your computing mind was off-line. How well can you expect to perform in this condition? When the body is being run by the stimulus/response mind, the person under the influence appears to be dumb, indecisive, and confused. He or she thinks this is normal behavior. Nothing makes sense to anyone but them. This is not the ability most people would want to portray on the golf course.

Now, how would you like to experience this restimulation when you're playing in a tournament? Want to make a great impression in front of your boss? Not when the stimulus/response mind is in action. Some people live in a constant state of partial or full shutdown and appear to be stupid or unable to learn or reason things out. However, barring some unfortunate damage to the brain, people in this condition are not really dumb. They are living in a constant state of restimulation, and they never have full use of their computing, analytical minds. We see this condition in young students who cannot absorb data or duplicate their lessons—and along comes some doctor to quickly prescribe some drug. This is not the answer. Remember, the mechanics of this shutdown are partial or full unconsciousness. So, if an individual's computing mind is shut down, they will experience some form of emotional unconsciousness, or feel physically uncomfortable, or not like themselves. This happens instantaneously, without the individual's consent or knowledge. It's very difficult to do anything, especially play golf in this condition.

Can anyone be expected to perform in life under this scenario, particularly if they live in an area filled with restimulators! Their conduct would vary from moment to moment. In a single day, they could go from feeling love to experiencing rage, or drop from exhilaration into depression or apathy. It is no wonder most recreational golfers consider the game a hopeless case. With the wide variety of conduct that can occur when the stimulus/response mind is in control, there may be sanity today and hopelessness tomorrow. Look around you. Out on the golf course there is confusion, indecision, and frustration, all in the name of "Why can't I?" Ah—but who really can play well if the "everything-equals-everything" mind is running the show? Do you think any golfer given the correct data would actually not be able to play well? It would be impossible not to.

The computing mind, in its purest sense, just has data, and it understands perfectly well how to analyze any situation given the correct information. After all, it is nothing more than a computer. Your computing mind is pure, rational, and will respond accurately based on its education and viewpoints. However, we are living in a world filled with moronic minds that can't compute important survival data. It's a world filled with whirlpools of confusion, mis-emotion, and egos. The stimulus/response mind, as you have seen, is totally destructive and may kick in at any time. Are you still confused as to why your golf game is inconsistent?!!

MORE WACKY BEHAVIOR PATTERNS

Have you ever noticed the range rat who hits amazingly well on the practice range before the game, but for some reason cannot carry it to the first tee? This is why. Typically, if we make a mistake, we automatically justify it with some kind of statement or excuse. We go on about the incident, explaining that it happened "because of" this or "because of" that. The mind feels it must do this in order to assure its own survival. It needs to protect the body by making sure that its computations are correct, no matter how wacky they might be. If you can't confront errors head-on, playing your optimum golf game is impossible. Learning how to correct mistakes is beyond reach.

It should be understood that these wacky behavior patterns are simply old survival patterns that once worked to solve problems. The stimulus/response mind (in which everything equals everything) believes that the same situation equals the same solution. The acting-out of a solution can take the form of any action. (We discuss these mind wars in Chapter 5.)

Take Bill and Fred, for example. Bill and Fred are playing a round of golf. Bill outplays Fred. Fred loses, and his computing mind shuts down. His stimulus/response mind kicks in, and the recorded message is, *Bill won. You lost.* Therefore, Bill's actions and words are recorded as being of greater survival value than Fred's, and the next time a similar situation occurs, Fred will become Bill. He will act, say, and literally "be" Bill to solve the problem. A personality shift occurs. You may have observed someone you know appear to change personalities as a situation changes. This may have even happened to you. This shift is a remnant survival personality that was adopted during pain or displeasure over a perceived loss. In order to survive, you *became* the winner by adopting their personality. This mechanism worked just fine when ancient people lived in caves, but as the primitive brain gave way to a more sophisticated one, this stimulus/response mind and its conclusions for surviving became madness. You can't play golf if you're not being you!

Want some more madness? How about those voices in your head? We all have them. They're the voices that talk to you, urging you to do something, criticizing you, demanding obedience. These voices can keep any, or many, of the senses from knowing reality. They are nothing more than hypnotic-like suggestions that are implanted or wired into your stimulus/response mind from the times when your analytical mind shut down. We call this phenomenon "mind noise." Mind noise is created during incidents of physical pain and emotional trauma, loss, or disappointment. You put those voices there. First, they came as an idea about how you can justify your action, then this idea attached itself to a mental picture, which reacted on your endocrine (hormonal) system to cause emotion. If you play golf with emotion, you're playing with a lot of effort. Effort involves force. You can't force golf. You play golf. Simply, play.

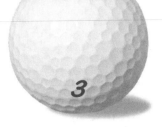

The Mind/Body Slump

*T*he loss of ability, as well as the inability to use your full potential as a golfer, is due to the mind/body slump. What is this, you ask? Simply put, it is a metabolic condition where the mind and body are working at less than optimum levels, usually against each other. This condition occurs when the mind seems to shut off, and the body runs on automatic. In this state, the stimulus/response mind is in control. It doesn't think. It runs on past experiences and cannot contemplate present or future situations. This is a less than desirable state, because the body is running totally off its environment, meaning everything that can happen to you will happen—not good on the golf course.

There was a time, however, when the mind of our early ancestors, at its purest, had great command over the body, and the body would carry out with precision everything the mind would command. However, through time and evolution, much of this ability was lost. The mind today is often in a state where it is less in command but rather running on automatic. It is very difficult to affect change, when the body-mind, which is designed to resist change, is in charge. When this happens, you can slide into a mind/body slump. You start operating at a lower level of metabolic efficiency, all along believing that you're performing optimally. This is one of life's greatest illusions. You think you're in control, but you're not. How can you perform that perfect swing if you're only partially conscious?

HOW THE SLUMP AFFECTS ABILITY AND PERFORMANCE

When in this slump, you're unable to demonstrate your skills with any level of proficiency. Tasks seem hard to accomplish. Things just don't seem to go right. You feel tired. You lose your drive and ambition, and your very zest for life suffers. When this biochemical condition occurs, you believe this condition is really you. It is not. Being in the slump allows the endocrine system to dictate emotions and moods to the nervous system. (Your hormones, along with the nervous system, control the body. They regulate almost all functions.) Remember, your body runs on automatic with one goal—to survive. If the collective cells of the body feel the mind is incapable of directing its survival, then the stimulus/response mind will take over, utilizing the nervous and hormonal systems to take whatever action is necessary to survive. This guy or gal does not know golf. You do. You are not your body. You just use one to play with while you're here in this universe.

You see, basically, the body is simply a machine. All the system's organs and cells are part of its vast machinery. This machine can run on automatic, or it can be controlled through the use of your mind. When you're in a slump, your life is literally up for grabs. You're no longer in the driver's seat. You're just a passenger hoping to stop and start in the right places and at the right times to collect the bounties of life. When you're out of the slump, you're in the driver's seat. You're in control, making all the right decisions, making all the right turns, collecting all that life has to offer. Using the mind allows you access to the full range of your skills and abilities.

This is a far better way to play golf than leaving your game up to data that has been collected and filed by the body. Some of these automatic mechanisms aren't so productive or golf positive. The mind receives data through the senses and defers action to the body. If you're not there that day, or your mind is not in present time, then the body will interpret that incoming data based on some past incident and not on data collected in the present. If you can observe something fully, you can understand it and demonstrate it. This is the essence of fully understanding the golf course and what action to take accordingly.

Playing a game of golf while you're in a slump creates an endless abyss of problems, frustration, missed opportunities, and a sense of hopeless-ness. When you're out of the slump and yourself, your game is great. Everything goes right, and you can't seem to do anything wrong. Your energy is boundless. Ideas flow through your mind, and you feel unstop-pable. You have luck, a love for life and living, and your performance on the golf course is masterful. Difficult shots become easier. Your reality levels soar. The ball looks larger. The greens are closer, and the cup seems wider. You don't necessarily have fewer problems, but you can handle them with more ease. Tiredness, fatigue, and weakness become things of the past. Fat loss and muscle tone become a natural thing, and strength is a given. Optimum health is easier to attain. When the body is doing its job and the mind is doing its job, you'll feel a great sense of command over your game. All these attributes indicate that you are out of the slump and performing at peak levels. Basically, you are in present time, operating in the future. Isn't golf a game of future time and space? Where the ball goes is the future, right? Right.

It may be a surprise to you, but these peak levels should be your normal state of living and playing. They only seem amazing because you're so used to being in the slump. Your good golf game is your normal golf game, and scores yet unheard of (for example, sub-sixties) would then be considered amazing.

TAKING CONTROL

Well, then, how do you stay out of this mind/body slump? It is a question that has been asked for centuries. Athletes, doctors, scientists, wise men, religious leaders, and society in general have all searched the ends of the earth for the solution. Actually, the answer is quite simple. Life is a constant balance between many factors, including the physical and the mental, power and knowledge, knowing and not knowing. There is a state of supreme balance between the body and the mind that pushes all else aside. A strong mind and a strong body are equally important. For optimum efficiency, they must work in tandem. A weakness in either side produces a condition of overall weakness.

There is only one true way to clear a path out of the maze of confusion and frustration and escape the slump—that is on the back of physical and mental power. To take back the power of your mind, you must begin by balancing the body's chemistry. Restoring homeostasis (a term used to describe a state of harmony between the interrelated functions and elements of the body) will allow the body to surrender its governing control. Then you will see and play golf with incredible clarity, talent, skill, and ability.

A golfer's physical and mental ability on the course depends on seven major factors: endurance, muscular strength, reaction time, agility, mobility, perception, and purpose. The quality and quantity of each of these factors adds up to a golfer's individual total ability. Although it is true that we are all born with certain pre-existing levels of each element, both practice and physical exercise greatly influence their development. A golfer's skill depends on his or her willingness to carry out his or her purpose without compromise. A golfer's determination can bring out the level of innate talent he or she possesses. It is our goal to help you balance these factors as best as possible. Achieving this goal will produce a calming effect on the mind, eliminating mind noise and letting your talent show through. That is what talent is. An individual who can come close to balancing all these factors has talent; the higher the degree of balance, the greater the talent.

Correct forms of exercise will enhance not only the physical factors mentioned (endurance, muscular strength, agility, and mobility), but also the mental factors (perception, purpose, and reaction time) by producing a calm in the mind via the body. This is ideal for the game of golf. Only when you apply force to the body will you free the mind.

Golf is a game of observing the obvious. When you quiet the mind noise, all of life goes still so that you can observe it fully, attack it totally, and push forward to the ultimate Atomic Golf experience. Mind noise can be controlled and conquered by confronting it first, knowing what it is— the echoes of past solutions to problems revisited—getting the body to relax, and then eliminating the body noise filtering into the mind. The body's chemistry, when out of balance due to a poorly conditioned body, will be very noisy. (With the use of the Atomic Golf techniques featured in later chapters, you will learn how to take back control of your mind and overcome this biochemical condition.)

An unconditioned body has to work harder to accomplish basic tasks. Breathing becomes labored. The heart has to pump harder and more often. The digestive tract is clogged, causing indigestion. The liver is less able to filter toxins and screams for help. The kidneys are under constant duress. Joints and connective tissues ache, and muscles are fatigued. These negative conditions are processed in the brain and filtered through the mind. As they flow from body to mind, they are constantly communicating and asserting their presence, mostly on a level undetectable to you, and they will throw off your game in a hurry, jamming your ability and performance. The constant noise interferes with decision-making processes that are critical on the golf course, especially when playing an important hole. However, when the body is finely tuned, much like a finely tuned car engine, and you can barely hear it running. Fine tune the body and you'll perform incredibly, with a calm mind, void of any internal noise pollution.

Your performance and ability on the golf course are directly related to your ability to keep your body and mind calm and in present time. A strong body, made fit and enduring, will resist the mind noises better, thereby allowing for a calm mind and an accurate assessment of time and space.

How does athletic performance or skill relate to time and space? Time and space are kissing cousins. One depends on the other for its existence. Time is everywhere, and yet it is nowhere. It is only perceived because you believe in it. By the time you perceive the present, it has already become the past. In order to truly operate in present time, at least where your golf game is concerned, you must perceive the future. If you learn a skill, the long drive, for example, and if you park that skill in a space of another time—a moment, even a parcel of time—you will not be able to perform that skill fully, for it has been left behind.

Therefore, ability, skill, and performance depend on the willingness to duplicate with certainty that skill or ability in present time.

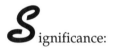

Perfect Mind:
The Nature of Failure and
the Inability to Succeed

*S*ignificance:

- *Webster's* **definition:** Importance; giving meaning to something.

- **Michalik/Manavian's definition:** Significance is worthless, extra, and unnecessary information. Separate from information you've believed. Example: golfer blames everything else for why he didn't hit correctly, except the real reason. As significances build up in the mind from life and living, the potential for logic is reduced, and illogical results occur. All failure, loss, "cannots," and "will nots" are due to agreed-upon significances. A person can be and can accomplish anything. Only their own false considerations doom them to failure. It starts with a violation of integrity—a state of unbroken wholeness, of moral principle and character, of truth and untainted virtue, even in the face of adversity. The person knows they can do something, but nevertheless they fail to act. This leads to committing acts that either agree with, or help convince them of, the fact they can't perform, which, of course, leads to the inability to act. They then take on the personality of a victim. This is not truly them. So now we have a person who isn't really himself or herself, thus putting them in a state of confusion, which leads to more problems. Overwhelmed, this person will respond with some action that is non-survival oriented and nonproductive. An individual in this state is not living in present time. They are in some kind of a daydream, acting out life. How can anyone be successful if they're not really present?

THE SOURCE OF ALL TALENT AND ABILITY

The mind is engaged in perceiving and remembering data, understanding problems, and formulating conclusions. The ability to perceive and retain data, to make conclusions, and to solve problems is directly related to overcoming mind noise and fully using the mind without the organism's interferences. As you have seen, the ultimate penalty of the body's involvement in the mind's affairs is stupidity, aberration, and pain.

Failure to use your analytical mind lowers your potential to succeed. Success in using your mind raises your ability and intelligence, thus moving you toward success—success in achieving the ultimate Atomic Golf swing. Both ability and intelligence are necessary if you are to obtain and persist at a high skill level. The worth of an individual in terms of their ability to succeed is judged on their ability to lessen the mind noise and make full use of their mind.

ACCEPTING INFORMATION

Your understanding of the golf swing is stored in the mind and utilized by the body. The mind, as we've said, is comparable to a computer. The mind plays the role of the information gatherer (software). The brain acts as a processor. The body acts as the operating system, on which you can run your individual software programs. Golf is simply a software program, just like walking, talking, or any other motor skill.

The reason you don't play to your ultimate mind potential as a golfer is because one or more of these components is being corrupted by false incoming data and not operating at maximum potential. Operating systems and software that have glitches in them do not execute properly and hence "crash."

Now, as a user of this system, your responsibility lies solely in understanding exactly how every one of these components works and interrelates with one another. This process of understanding requires using information for the specified areas of the mind, body, and golf.

Unfortunately, there is a vast sea of information available to anyone who is attempting to learn anything. There is more information on golf and fitness than any other sport on this planet, yet the golfing population consists of overweight hacks who can't break one hundred! How is this possible? The reason is simple: all of this information cannot be utilized unless it is understood and its value demonstrated. The data must be categorized before use for maximum benefit. The brain separates information into the following categories:

- vital information
- missing information
- false information
- altered information
- contrary information
- inapplicable information

Whatever information you agree with (in other words, agreed-upon significances that you accept) is what you program in, and therefore it is exactly what you will perform. The information given here on the mind, body, and golf swing is just the vital and relevant information you need. If you accept certain information that is false on the golf swing, then you will continue to perform based on that false information and will crash at some point short of your ultimate goal.

With this Atomic Golf System, we can actually say that the action of hitting a golf ball is a simple and a learnable task that anyone can develop. This is contrary to the standard belief held by both golfers and nongolfers who think that hitting a golf ball is an extremely difficult task and impossible to master. What are the core elements that have lead you to failure? We will explore this and much more in the next two chapters. The trick is to see through all the muck, confusion, and false data so that what is valuable may be revealed and recorded.

Just the fact that you bought and are reading this book is a step in the right direction. Continue on this journey and you will reap the benefits of the Atomic Golfer.

ABILITY LOST AND FOUND

What is ability, and why does it come and go? In our case, we're dealing with golf skills. How come, after you have mastered a particular swing or putt, you cannot duplicate it each time? Taking into consideration variables in the environment, humans, like no other creature, have the ability to concentrate on a single thought for as long as it takes to develop a skill. Why then, only from time to time, is this skill demonstrable, and you cannot remember those thoughts and memory of your learned skill? Why do people go into slumps? What happens to this ability, where does it go? Does it leave and decide to come back? A skill once learned correctly should always be available, like a command in a software program. It is locked in the mind to be retrieved. Why is it not always retrievable? It seems to be covered over or misplaced. It is because factors like mind noise, mis-thoughts, mis-emotions, and not-thereness (a state in which someone is not operating in present time; rather, they are in sort of a not-recognizable daydream) make those skills irretrievable, and thus unable to be demonstrated. Hard to believe but undeniably true.

The mind/body slump has affected many players. Slumps usually occur in the beginning of tournaments or near the end on championship Sundays. We have compiled a list of some notable incidents, not to rehash these moments for the players, but rather to validate how and why it could occur with anyone not in ultimate mental and physical condition.

T. C. Chen

Taiwanese golfer T. C. Chen had played magnificently for the first three days of the 1985 U.S. Open at Oakland Hills, setting fifty-hole tournament records with his play. Playing the fifth hole, he was around the green in two and faced a simple chip shot. With everything going his way up until this point, Chen unbelievably decelerates his club as it passes under the ball then attempts to recover by accelerating post impact and actually hits his ball twice during one shot. Chen makes an unthinkable quadruple bogey eight on that hole and hands the tournament to Andy North by a shot!

Tiger Woods

Fast-forward eleven years to 1996. Tiger Woods has the main stage at the U.S. Open, again being played at Oakland Hills. Playing only in his second U.S. Open, Tiger at age twenty is still an amateur and a student at Stanford University. He began round one by grabbing the spotlight as he started his opening round in a blaze. Scorching the front nine, with highlights that included holing his third shot from the fairway on the fourth hole, then hitting the stick with his second shot on the very next hole, and after a birdie on twelve, he is actually tied for the lead at two under par. Mysteriously, all of a sudden, starting on the fourteenth hole, he proceeds to go bogey, double bogey, quad, and bogey, to fall off the leader board, and shoot a disappointing seventy-six for the day. The height of this collapse came on the sixteenth hole. Off the tee, in perfect position, he hit his second shot into the water guarding the green. He then proceeded to take a penalty stroke and a drop, then dumped it into the water yet again. After another penalty and drop, he hit his ball, two putting for an eight. Tiger went on to shoot seventy-six that day and eventually ended the tournament in a tie for eighty-second place. What could have possibly happened to him? What gave out? How could a player of his caliber, who was in fact playing at the top of his game during the most stressful of conditions, collapse like this?

Arnold Palmer

From 1958 to 1964, Arnold Palmer dominated golf, earning the nickname "The King" and attracting thousands of adoring fans who were dubbed "Arnie's Army." In that span, he won his seven major championships: four Masters, two British Opens, and one U.S. Open. Those victories were memorable, but Palmer also was capable of memorable—make that spectacular—losses.

No loss was more spectacular than his back nine collapse at the 1966 U.S. Open at the Olympic Club in San Francisco. Not only did he have what seemed an insurmountable lead, but he also had a chance to break Ben Hogan's Open record score of 276 over seventy-two holes. Palmer led Billy Casper by three shots before the final round. Palmer, homing in on Hogan's record, shot a brilliant thirty-two on the front nine and had a seven-shot lead on Casper as they teed off on the tenth. Palmer made bogey on the tenth hole, but it was no cause for concern because he had a six-shot lead with eight holes to play. That lead held up through the next two holes, with each man going par-birdie. Palmer then missed the green on the thirteenth to make another bogey, his lead cut to five. But instead of closing the deal on Casper, he was thinking about Hogan's record. If he could finish the last five holes in par, he would break the record by a shot.

Both players made par on the fourteenth, but Palmer bogeyed the next three holes, allowing Casper to pull even with two birdies and a par. Each made par on the eighteenth, sending the championship to an eighteen-hole playoff that Casper won, sixty-nine to seventy-three. How could Arnold Palmer, the same man who came back from a seven-stroke deficit in the final round of the 1960 U.S. Open, now give away seven strokes? Why didn't he go seven more under and win by fourteen? What was it that changed The King's ability down the stretch?

Phil Mickelson and Craig Stadler

Back at the 2002 Players Championship, former Masters champion Craig Stadler and two-time major champion Phil Mickelson both experienced the mind/body slump for all to see on national television.

Craig Stadler had a stretch of holes on the back nine at the TPC Sawgrass that went birdie/birdie/ace/par/birdie, placing him within a shot of the lead. He promptly followed this unconscious display with a horrific finish that went bogey, double bogey, triple bogey. Meanwhile, Phil was two shots off the lead when he chipped onto the tenth hole and was staring down an eighteen-foot putt for par. He knocked it past five feet, missing the comeback. He then proceeded to miss the comeback's comeback from another five feet, leaving two feet that he then missed again!!! When the dust settled, he five-putted the green, going from a potential par/bogey at worst to a quadruple bogey, and destroying any and all chances of winning the tournament. How is it possible that moments like these can occur? These are supposed to be the best players in the world, aren't they?

Greg Norman

Undoubtedly, there is no pro golfer who has suffered more torturous losses at the brink of victory than Greg Norman. In 1986, he led every major championship of the year going into the final round, yet he won only one of those four tournaments. In the 1986 PGA Championship, he watched helplessly as Bob Tway blasted his ball into the cup from a greenside bunker on the seventy-second hole to claim the title. A year later, at the Masters, Norman endured even more heartbreak when Larry Mize holed out a forty-five-yard chip to win in sudden death. That should have been enough for any mortal to bear, but there were more tournaments to follow. He lost the 1990 Nestle Invitational on Robert Gamez's winning last hole, a 176-yard eagle. One month later, with Norman watching, "The Shark" sank when David Frost belted his ball out of a bunker and into the cup on the last hole of the USF&G Classic for a tournament-winning birdie.

But nothing compared to the agony of the 1996 Masters. During the first two rounds, Norman played incredible, shooting rounds of sixty-three to sixty-nine, and gaining a four-stroke lead over Nick Faldo. Norman was playing far better than anyone that week in extraordinary conditions of high winds and concrete-hard greens. With the field stroke average of 74.3, Norman was one of only seven golfers to shoot in the sixties. That Saturday, Norman was paired with Faldo and shot a one under seventy-one to open up a six-shot lead over Faldo.

Norman was playing like a man of destiny. This coveted title had eluded Norman since his best chance in 1986, when a charging forty-six-year-old Jack Nicklaus shot a final-round sixty-five, combined with Norman's ill-fated five-iron that flew right off the entire sixty-yard gallery on the eighteenth hole, leading to a bogey that lost the tournament by a shot. On the final day, it seemed impossible for him to lose as he was threatening to break all sorts of records. Norman started off badly and hit his opening shot into the trees. It was a sign of things to come. He hit only three of the first nine greens, bogeying the first, fourth, and ninth holes while birdying only the second. Faldo nailed three birdies and suffered only one bogey. With only nine holes left to play, Norman's six-shot lead was down to two.

He missed a ten-foot par putt on number ten after missing the green left. Then he three-putted number eleven, missing the par putt from thirty inches. On number twelve, for the second day in a row, Norman left his tee shot short into Rae's Creek. While he was able to recover for a great bogey on Saturday, this time he made a double-bogey five.

Faldo was content to make pars during this stretch and pulled ahead by two. Both players birdied the two par fives, numbers thirteen and fifteen. Then Norman relinquished any chance he had of winning when he hit into the water on the par three, sixteenth hole.

Faldo finished his fabulous day by making a birdie on number eighteen for a final round of sixty-two to Norman's seventy-eight (scores in each of the four rounds: 63-69-71-78 = 281). How could one of the greatest golfers of all time, who had won so many tournaments, and who had a six-shot lead at a course on which he had the course record, collapse as severely as Norman did here? What changed? What went wrong? People have agreed that the back nine on Sunday at a major championship is difficult. Why wasn't he better prepared for it? Why couldn't he fix it?

Jean Van de Velde

The 1999 British Open Championship held at Carnoustie Golf Links was one of the most difficult British Opens of recent time. Frenchman Jean Van de Velde had meticulously played the course in great fashion. He led the field in putting the entire week and seemed to be coasting through the entire tournament. With seventy-one holes completed and a three-shot lead, the engraver had literally started putting his name on the coveted Claret Jug trophy. All that was left for the Frenchman was the 418 yards of the final hole—a straightforward hole that paralleled the first hole, with water both to the right and at seventy yards short of the green. Jean blocked his tee shot so far to the right that it actually went over the water and onto a small peninsula shaped piece of land that belonged to the first hole. Visibly shaken, he could have easily pitched out ninety yards and had a simple shot left from one hundred yards, put it on the green, and even if he had taken as many as four putts, he would still have won. Instead, he hit a two-iron way to the right, which sailed over the creek, hitting the very top post of the grandstands, ricocheting back toward him, bouncing off the rock wall guarding the creek that it had just cleared, and ending up some twenty-five yards short of the creek.

Left with no more than 160 yards to the green, playing out of two-foot-tall grass, Van de Velde mis-hit his shot and landed in the creek. From there, he debated about playing the shot out of the water. He even took off his shoes and socks to the approval of the drunken Scottish crowd. However, the creek bed rose and covered his ball further. Forced to take relief from the water, playing his fifth shot, he was faced with playing a similar shot from tall grass. With the flag tucked on the right side of the green and well guarded by a sand bunker, he short-sided himself and hit into the bunker! His competitor, Craig Parry from Australia, was a foot away from Jean's ball in the bunker in two shots and holed his shot for a birdie three! Van de Velde, seeing that he needed to do the same for the British Open Championship, hit his shot fifteen feet past the cup. Needing the putt for a triple bogey seven to just get into a three-way playoff, miraculously, he drained it. The Frenchman's topsy-turvy play continued for the four-hole play-off, which he lost to Englishman Paul Lawrie.

Interesting to note that one hole left to play, just 418 measly yards, was all that separated Van de Velde from the championship. He had unquestionably played far superior to anyone else in the field that week. Yet when it came down to enduring the final test of the seventy-two holes, he tanked. How could this happen? Why did this happen? How could it be prevented in the future?

STEP OUT FROM THE SHADOW

It is incidents like these that have caused practice fairways to be worn out with no resolution, driven expert technicians of the game mad, or led others to seek solace on the bar stool. But truly, the very best of these "slumpers" end up in the broadcast booths so they may point out everyone else's slumps. Yet the questions asked here have never been answered thoroughly enough, which is proved by the mere fact that these incidents keep repeating themselves—to the extent that it is now considered normal operation for golfers. Mark Calcavecchia set the lowest seventy-two-hole total of all time, then missed the cut the very next week! The Atomic Golfer will not have any weaknesses or uncontrollable variables—no highs and lows—as they will not be tolerated. Supplant the current success rate for golfers as the new standard. He or she will be a wrecking ball on the golf course.

In conclusion, it is crystal clear that without the ability to totally focus and concentrate on the task at hand, you will never step out of the shadow of a slump. Techniques for dealing with a slump will be revealed in Chapter 6.

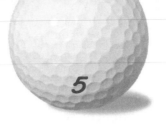

5

Mind Wars

*H*ave you ever hit a ball too far over or way short of the green? Or have you hit it the right distance, but just a few yards off line? You probably blamed your swing, as 99.9 percent of all golfers do, when in fact, your swing was executed properly. The error occurred because you were fed the wrong information. The information gathered was wrong because you weren't completely in present time to be able to see the data! An inability to observe the obvious is the major factor that leads to gathering misinformation such as bad yardage, wrong clubs, and so forth, which all leads to the proper execution of the wrong information. Though the golf swing is ultimately important, as you'll learn in Part Three, it should not be the first thing you look at. Golf is a difficult enough game for anyone to master while being fully conscious, but nearly impossible for those in a state of unconsciousness.

So how do you get into this out-of-present-time scenario? When did it all start, what causes it, and what can you do about it? Well, let's take a look at what's involved.

EVERYWHERE ELSE BUT HERE

When it comes to building the human brain and body, all the construction materials are available in our DNA. The Who, What, When, Where, and Why of the brain and mind has remained largely a mystery. But a lot of the mystery has been worked out. Studies suggest that the inner workings of the mind are formed and determined, in large part, by events that occur in the environment. The other two influences are toxins and stress. It has been suggested that our early childhood, even prebirth, experiences determine our brain's emotional stability and calculating powers. It seems that the brain wires and rewires itself from these experiences on a kind of feedback mechanism. The sights, sounds, smells, and sensations associated with these experiences can determine how we act and perceive things later on in life. This we believe to be true, but there is another consideration much more sinister in nature. It's the secret of your DNA and how it retains data from your parents, their parents, and so on down the line.

It is a recognized fact that you inherit your physical traits, skills, and abilities. But you also inherit all the good and bad data from the minds of your ancestors. Everything your parents did, their parents did, and so forth has been recorded and stored as data, and it is forever present in your DNA. Positive and negative thoughts, healthy and destructive emotions, rational and irrational fears and phobias, and so on, interact to make a composite of you, your inherited DNA, and the world around you. Furthermore, research in quantum physics (a branch of science that studies the behavior of matter and energy at its smallest level) has shown that pain can produce computer-like viruses that can cloud a person's ability to think and know (knowingness). All data is stored in mental pictures in the stimulus/response mind—either while you're conscious or unconscious. These mental pictures contain energy. This energy acts upon the nervous system—good or bad. Some of these unpleasant moments can get restimulated, or reenacted, at any time, whether it's a day, a month, even years later.

One survival mechanism the mind uses to protect itself from these painful memories, or to escape an existence or experience that has become too painful, is to remove itself temporarily from present time. The experience is similar to daydreaming or wandering off somewhere in your mind. We've all observed these lapses in others and experienced them ourselves. They can even happen at a profoundly deep level, beyond your awareness and at unpredictable times, such as when you're trying to make that crucial putt or long drive in an important golf outing.

THE EFFECTS OF BEING ELSEWHERE

Being out-of-present time is the chief cause of all mishaps and accidents. Accidents happen when your awareness is compromised so you make a mistake, or you are not alert enough to handle another's mistakes. When you are fully there . . . here! Now! You're it. You would never stub your toe, bump your head, or drop that glass if you were alert and in present time. The same is true in sports. Someone who is fully present, can and will, at that moment, demonstrate his or her skill or talent to their fullest. The less present they are in the here and now, the less they can demonstrate.

This failure, so to speak, of the mind to stay analytically stable, balanced, and present affects the emotions, thus affecting your biochemistry, mainly the endocrine system (hormones), which influences the body's muscular and nervous systems. Neuromuscular ability is responsible for carrying out that golf swing. Yes, your golf swing! These emotions may feel like normal behavior. Sometimes, if your knowingness is highly developed, you will feel something is not quite right, but you can't put your finger on it. And you truly can't! It's hidden under countless layers of life, living, and mis-emotion. It sure will mess up your golf game, and it can happen at a moment's notice. Witness all the great golfers from the last chapter who, for some reason unbeknownst to them, crashed their games out of nowhere. We have all seen it time after time, in every other sport.

However, the opposite is also true. When an athlete or player makes an incredible score, hit, catch, basket, or other astonishing sports play, it's seen as a superhuman feat. The skill of the person in that event, which seemed to be far beyond everyone else's ability, is just an example of a normal play from someone who (with great skill) could stay in the present long enough to demonstrate it.

Without going into fancy physics terms and the like, we will simply give you the basic facts based upon our discussion of not-thereness or subtle daydreaming and explain how this can affect you. As touched upon earlier, time and space are related. Space is where you are "at." You are in this space, and time positions you here. In the past, you were in that space at that past time. In the future, you will be in some future place. That place will be your time to be there.

In present time, you are in a space, let's say on a golf course, on the eighth green at noon—this is your present time, your present space. However, let's say that for some reason unbeknownst to you, your game starts to go badly. Out of nowhere, things just begin going wrong. When this happens, a restimulation of some memory, small or large, real or imaginary, has taken your mind out of present time and placed it in this restimulation, sending you into another time and space. Sure, your body's there, but your mind's not. You're not there to operate the machinery—your body. This restimulation could be caused by anything—a person, a phrase, a smell, the cold, the heat. All the senses record incidents, and anything that reminds you of an incident will bring it up for viewing by your mind. Meanwhile, while you're viewing these restimulations, your golf game is going by the boards.

Sounds fantastic, doesn't it? But it's true, and it has been proven countless times. Any subtle change in biochemistry brought about by the mind playing tricks on you is a disaster to your golf game. Come on, you've heard countless sports broadcasters remarking that a certain guy is in a "funk" or "slump" or something of the like, then saying he just has to go through it and he'll recover. Generally speaking, they do. They will eventually come back to themselves. The length of time this takes is dependent on a player's lifestyle. A cleaner life brings about change sooner, as opposed to a not-so-clean life, which will take much longer. The procedure called In the Moment on page 62 provides a method of handling these moments.

We all desire success, whether it's success in life or on the golf course. You have the potential to take charge of your life, thus bringing into focus the full power and skills you possess. The problem is, if you never figure out why and how you got into this mindless state, you are certainly doomed to return to it sooner or later. Your golf game becomes a rollercoaster ride.

MAJOR CONTRIBUTORS TO NOT-THERENESS

All of us experience anger, fear, grief, and other troublesome emotions, but they only exist because we are unable to control them. These emotions and the negative energy they produce are some of the major contributors to not-thereness. It's important to develop a greater perspective by looking at situations from all angles. If you look at only one aspect of a situation, you will produce a solid mind, keeping all of your mind's energies locked in a ball. This mind-ball keeps thoughts swirling around in your head in a random figure-this, figure-that, bouncing thoughts off each other. It will create confusion and emotion and cause us to look inside our heads for solutions to problems—but the solution only exists when you look outward at what is really happening. On the golf course, these troublesome emotions will not allow you to use your skill correctly.

In order to progress through the Atomic Golf System, you will need to understand the following viewpoints and ideas about mis-emotions and negative energy and how they trigger a variety of mechanisms and scenarios that take you out of present time.

The "I Can't-Be-Wrong" Mechanism

Our day-to-day emotional pressures and stresses often end up with us on the golf course. For example, an individual may be suffering from some life-related problems—say a difficulty with a significant other or spouse, alcohol, money, or so on. He goes to the golf course to work on his swing. He's thinking about the mortgage payments or his wife's birthday, and then all of a sudden—poof! A bad swing. There may be nothing wrong with his swing, but there is definitely something wrong with his ability to cope or deal with his thoughts. The mind controls the body, which is basically mechanical. If your mind is elsewhere, or has its attention on some other thought, then your golf will suffer. Your swing becomes mechanical. Any kind of uncertainty will destroy your statistics on the course.

As previously explained, these mind blocks create an emotional curve and do their nasty deeds to the muscular and nervous systems, thus affecting your swing, and you can't figure out what is happening. You will look and ponder and figure this and that all for nothing. The mind will make up all sorts of excuses, never really getting to the cause. You see, the mind has to come up with some acceptable conclusion for its inability to perform because the mind believes its viewpoints are infallible. Failure is nonsurvival, and your mind can't have that!

The mind has a self-preservation mechanism. It is created in such a way to think that it can never be wrong. This self-preservation mechanism was developed through evolution to preserve our survival. But this once-useful mechanism is now a curse. Now, we all feel we have to be right about things—right about admitting wrong, right about being wrong, right about doing wrong. Your mind will not accept that you made a bad, nonsurvival judgment or act. The mind is programmed not to make a mistake, but the parts under the influence of the body-mind or stimulus/response mind do. So your mind wrestles with this debate, "How I can make a mistake is not in my program" verses "it's nonsurvival and it will kill me if I admit it." You rationalize and justify being right. This is the basis of all arguments and bad decisions. On the golf course, this mechanism will prevent you from making a real decision based on facts, not emotions, causing bad swings and worse putts. Just being aware of this "can't-be-wrong" mechanism will go a long way toward keeping your mind and emotions stable.

Remember, this outdated, worn-out mechanism of being right is not necessary anymore. It's all right to admit wrongdoings as long as you acknowledge them with responsibility. If someone tries to make you wrong, just acknowledge their viewpoint and don't argue the point. It is pointless!

Alternate Identities

People sometimes are not themselves. They take on the personalities of others. These alternate identities are a primary cause of sonic, visual, and body shutoffs. This is the guy in the slump—that funk. He just can't seem to get his skills going, and he's right! He can't because he isn't there! He stays locked away in the back of his mind while some alternate takes his place.

You look at this guy and say, "Oh my gosh, what happened? Why can't he play golf today?" He can. His alternate can't. The alternate identity is a survival mechanism. It's one way the mind uses to escape a too-painful existence or experience. Often, you'll hear a player complain to herself, "I could kick myself for missing that putt!" or, "I just hate myself for not doing well." Actually, this is the primary mechanism that causes an individual to dislike himself or herself. She actually does not dislike herself at all, rather, she dislikes the alternate self she has been forced to become and thinks it's her.

These alternate identities are regulated by negative energy in the mind, which gets its power from doubt, fear, and other mis-emotions. When all is well, an individual can maintain himself or herself. There's little or no negative energy in the mind to cause this alternate shift. But as soon as the energy increases, the real guy or gal is less and less able to control the alternate. It all comes down to self-control. Self-control is the power exerted by self. It's integrity. If an individual has enough of integrity, then self-determination exists to the degree to which the self is able to command and control the moment. Mis-emotions open the door for alternates.

These alternate personalities are copies of anyone who is perceived as a winner, a survivor, in a nonsurvival situation. It could be a fictional character in a story, comic book, or movie. It could be the hero or the villain, a big brother, sister, friend, or even an enemy. It could be anyone who is perceived to have won. Therefore, we adopt their personalities, along with their habits and mannerisms—their identities. And, we adopt them unknowingly. It amounts to an individual losing confidence in self. So, in order to survive, you take on this alternate. It is not you, but is pretending to be or thinks it is.

Alternate personalities or egos can also move in when something or someone indicates you should be someone else. It can be caused by phrases like "Why can't you be more like your father, or brother, or uncle?" Another could be, "Hit the ball like Hogan or Palmer." These phrases imply that another's ability is greater and may cause you to shift. When this shift occurs, you are gone. Your ability to be in present time is gone. Your skills are diluted, and you can't figure out what's happening. Humans learn their first lessons, basic habits, mannerisms, and skills through mimicry. An alternate personality mimics someone who has demonstrated, in their life, a greater ability to complete a survival task than you.

This condition is your split or dual (athletic) personality. If the golfer is in good shape physically and emotionally, if they have strong self-control and integrity, coupled with a firm belief in themselves, then they will perform magnificently. But if they allow themselves to be restimulated by a real or imaginary nonsurvival situation, the golfer is doomed to failure, or at least to less than their optimal performance, while ironically adopting the "winning" personality.

Now, any professional who supposes to help this poor soul might wind up diagnosing them with every false condition imaginable, including compulsions, neuroses, obsessions and all the rest, missing the basic source of the problem. The cells evolved long ago, and evolution created this once-necessary survival mechanism to assure progress. But those cells have now grown into a human being, and this once-necessary mechanism is now his downfall. Being others is not being self.

The Speed of Life

Okay, let's look at the mind's ability to be present from the point of view of the speed of life. Who can reach it? Whoever has found the missing piece in the mystery of "Why can't I [blank] all the time"? Life is motion, isn't it? Well, let's look closer. Although life itself looks as if it's in motion, it is actually a multitude of still pictures moving so fast that it appears to be moving, just like a movie, which was derived from the term "motion pictures." (Bear with us here because this does relate to your golf.) Prove it to yourself. Look at a fan blade. Now, concentrate on just one blade. If you can, you will realize it goes still for just a nanosecond. All of life is stop and go. All you have to do is catch up with it, and you can control it. You know, control? How you get the ball in the hole, right? The closer you get to the speed of life, the more you'll be able to observe and the more control you'll have.

For example, let's take a putt. The ball isn't actually in constant motion, but rather it is in a series of stop-and-go frames. If you able to control each individual frame, you will be able to master where you want to locate the ball.

Another example of how still frames create the illusion of constant motion is if you are on a train platform and a speeding train goes by and you are asked to describe what the person in the third seat of the third car is wearing. You couldn't possibly because the train would be moving past you much too quickly (just like life is). However, if you were moving alongside the train at the same speed (for as certain physics tells us, life is not going to slow down), the better you would be able to look and observe. After all, that is what we're trying to do—to get you to be in the here and now so you can perceive accurately. If you are fully present, you will be able to perceive accurately, no matter how fast something is happening.

As we grow older and gather more information and experiences, we begin to lose focus. Things get cloudy and thick. This thickness slows your ability to perceive the speed of life accurately. It's similar to going for an eye exam and finding that some of the letters on the chart are out of focus. You may be able to read them, but it requires a lot of effort. The doctor moves you closer or puts a lens in front of you and those letters become clearer, sharper, and more defined. Well, most of us have been walking around out of focus our entire lives, performing in life with little horsepower. When you move into the nowness, the dimension of present time, your focus becomes crisp. You see things for what they are. Details and distances are easy and recognizable. The power, accuracy, and sheer will to deliver that little white ball exactly where you want it every time will be yours.

Life Is Energy—Good and Bad

Energy is the most powerful force in the universe. The mind's energy has no rival. Energy knows no boundaries, good or bad, evil or friendly. You can utilize the mind's energy for production or destruction. Life is energy. Golf consumes energy. All matter is made up of energy. It stands to reason that you should stay on the good side of energy and learn to channel it toward your goals.

The mind is very malleable. It can change instantly, simply if you miss a putt or drive a ball offline. In these moments, you must learn to leave all negative actions in the past. Look at your next shot in a new unit of time. Leave that bad shot in the past and move into the future. Calm the mind and save that energy for the next shot. Tolerance and patience are signs of strength.

It is important that you maintain your integrity, even in the face of adversity. It's important to engage golf with self-confidence (but also to avoid the negative qualities of conceit or arrogance). Never feel hopeless or demoralized. These negative emotions use up lots of energy from your cells, energy that you need to stay strong, fight off fatigue, and play a heck of a round of golf.

Contrary to what you might believe, the difficult times on the course, the mental and physical barriers you just can't seem to overcome, provide the best opportunity to gain useful insight and develop inner strength. It's strange but true; barriers are brothers to success. Every time you run into some golfing barrier, if you persist and don't break down (remember integrity), you will beat the barrier and play with greater success. Barriers are opportunities to get you to take a look and see what has just happened and formulate a plan to push forward, past the barrier.

After all, golf is a game, and what is a game? It is play versus stops. It is success versus barrier. It is "I want to" versus "No, I can't." The secret is that you *can*. If you persist, believe in yourself, stay in the now, and maintain integrity, you will win. Every time you win the mind war, you get stronger. You will be tested. Most fail or quit on some level. Life is a game. It is set up so you fail or else there would be no game. A win/win scenario is not a game. It's boring, and soon you would lose interest. So too is a lose/lose scenario. Fortunately, that is not the game of life or the game of golf. It's win some/lose some. That is what keeps the game going. Think about it. Isn't all of life like this? No barrier—no game.

So, don't be upset over a loss or barrier. Barriers create space and time. They give you the chance to reevaluate your game. Embrace them. If all the barriers were removed, we would eventually run out of space and then run out of time. Isn't this what happened to Elvis Presley? No more game, so he checked out. He simply ran out of things to do. He had no barrier left to overcome, so he became a victim of space and time. Relish the stops and bring them on. The wins become bigger. Your successes become greater. How many times have you seen someone retire from their job and the challenges of work, only to die shortly after? He or she simply ran out of play. No play, no life, no time. So bring on those long carries over water hazards, the tucked pin placements, and the impossible putts. Go right at them, and you know what? You'll not only play better, you'll also live longer. You are the hunter and the hunted. You control the outcome of either destiny. You set the traps of life and carry out your own execution. The only way through this maze of entrapment is the ability to recognize in present time what is before you.

Transgressions

A key part of any golfer's life is their ability to stay calm and keyed out (meaning detached yet present, not elsewhere) from their environment so they can fully concentrate on their efforts. In order to achieve this state, the golfer needs to understand what can prevent an optimum state of mind/body readiness. The following will give some insight into this condition.

Do you believe in karma, also called bad energy/good energy? Well, you should! For whatever name it is given, it's just a matter of physics. Energy once created cannot be destroyed, only altered. If you create bad energy, it will come back to its source, but with even greater force than originally exerted. Golfers need all the good karma and luck they can get. And luck is when hard work meets opportunity. Karma presents that opportunity.

If you commit transgressions against someone, some harmful or cruel act or deed, you will suffer from it at some point. If you commit transgressions against yourself, violating what you know or doing what you know you shouldn't, you will become a victim of some unpleasant act. If you do nothing when someone else commits transgressions, simply standing back and ignoring it, you will suffer. Transgressions against you that are ignored and not handled will double in pain and suffering.

You see, negative energy builds up in the cells of the body and is later dispersed in the nervous system. The nervous system then deposits this energy in the brain, where it affects the mind. Transgressions such as lies and other unethical behavior that are not handled wind up persisting in the mind, hidden away like some computer virus ready to cause all sorts of trouble for you in life—and most certainly on the golf course—when the pressure is on.

These old transgressions can, and will, reappear at any time and place. When they reappear, they are like a movie replaying its plot inside your head. The unconscious mind is the viewer. When it views this replay, it triggers your nervous system and endocrine system to kick in mis-emotions, indecision, and confusion. All this happens without your conscious awareness or permission. This whole scenario will take you out of present time. And how can you perform your best on a golf course if you're not all there?

Let's examine how these transgressions take hold of you. Here's how this happens. Let's say as a kid you hit someone with a bat and it hurt him. You took no responsibility for that incident at the time and forgot about it. It turns out that you grow up to be a baseball player. Everything is going fine and then, one day, out of the blue, some kid in the stands reminds you of the kid you hit many years before. This visual trigger will activate a mechanism in your mind, and that old incident will play itself out with full force in your unconscious. It will affect your nervous system and your endocrine system, sending you straight into the muck—into a slump. The greater the restimulation or duplication is, the greater the confusion and the stronger the mind/body slump.

Any golfer suffering from this cannot for the life of her figure out what went wrong. You see, these incidents are not for your conscious viewing. While you're trying to view the next green, your mind has got you looking at some past picture. Once you are able to key out, you can regain your ability and play well.

Any transgressions that you have committed in your past may cause this condition. Transgressions do not have to be physical; they can also be emotional. If you had a loss of some kind that really affected you, or you caused another person loss or misfortune, it may alter your ability to concentrate and perceive clearly. The procedure called Present Time Here and Now on page 61 will show you how to rid yourself of these past transgressions. So let's clean up all those old problems and refrain from committing new ones.

The Jungle Inside Your Head

Athletes in all sports have commented on how, during moments of good play, they were able to be "in the moment." They attributed good play to their ability to stay outside their heads and in the game. Therefore, this "moment" would seem to be a state outside of your thoughts that enhances your ability to focus on the game.

Any athlete will tell you that too much thinking can ruin any game. Thinking too much is a very dangerous game. As you've read in this chapter, the mind is filled with many traps, barriers, and aberrant viewpoints. Certainly, your abilities and skills can never be rekindled by looking for them inside your head. Your skills are there, programmed in. It's what you agree to on the golf course that determines your game.

If you look inside your head for the answers, you'll get more than you bargained for. There is so much junk mail in the mind in the form of mind viruses, but there is no spam blocker to protect you so you will just spin around in there. You will figure this and figure that, back and forth, spinning you deeper and deeper. It's like the mechanics of a computer. If you don't know how to access specific information, you're liable to get all sorts of extraneous information. It's the same with the mind. We are so used to the brain and mind working on automatic that we do not possess the skill to access what we really need to know. You question why you can't duplicate a good hit each time. If you're hitting it right, why aren't the same results being produced? It's your inability to access key data that's recorded and stored in the mind and coordinate that with what you observe on the golf course that fails you.

What you want to do is to get in touch with the environment, to see things as they truly are, to really look and be there. The key here is to notice the differences in things and how they really appear: the slope of the fairway to the flatness of the green; the direction of the wind to the calmness of the lake; the distance to the front of the green, and the distance to the flagstick. It is these differences that enhance your perception. This will separate things out and transform them from two- to three-dimensional objects. You'll play your best golf in three dimensions. Don't associate things with one another. See their differences. Good golfers play golf. Bad golfers, or the ones that go bad, think about the game while they're playing. Good golfers "know" while bad golfers try to "figure things out." Good golfers look out; bad golfers look inward. People in general just don't know how to look. Never look in. It's a trap. People are in a constant state of looking in— thinking. Rarely do they ever look out and truly see.

You can only see differences if you are truly there 100 percent of the time, outside your inner thoughts. Mistakes are made when we slide into the past or some other imaginary place. Not being in present time is like running out of gas in a drag race. The competition keeps going, but you can't catch up. Slowly, but surely, you're eventually so far behind that you lose momentum. Now your goals seem so far out of reach that many decide to give in. Don't be troubled, though. There is hope, read on!

Invalidations and Out-Points

Have you ever hit a bad shot and got caught up in it, or hit a great shot and invalidated yourself by calling yourself lucky? When you evaluate yourself, you are basically telling yourself what you think. Evaluation is defined as the act of accepting stable data without giving new or better data with which to agree. When you agree that you were lucky, you evaluate, or worse, invalidate your abilities. This raises doubt in the mind, which will set up a doubt circuit. The next time you come across a similar situation on the course, the doubt circuit will kick in and you will kick out.

Refuting, degrading, or discrediting something you know to be true is considered an invalidation. Anytime you deny yourself exactly what happened in a moment, you have, in effect, challenged your own knowingness. When this happens, it confuses your mind. You see it all the time on the golf tour. A player will birdie hole three and bogie holes four and five. Why? Most of the time, it's because he hoped he'd do well on the third hole, but didn't really believe he could do it. When the birdies occur, he feels relieved and kind of lucky. That sort of "half-I-can, half-I-hope-I-can" mentality will be reflected in his drives on holes four and five. It is best to recognize your shot only and move on without engaging the mind. You can talk about it later.

What is an out-point? *Webster's Dictionary* describes *out* as "away from, removed from a place, position, or situation"; also, "to remove from power." *Point* is defined as "geometrically having a definite position, precisely specified in nature"; also, as "a purpose or aim." An out-point, therefore, is to be removed from a definite position in space, a not-thereness. Being in a slump or not performing optimally are examples of out-points. When elsewhere, you are apt to misinterpret data in any of the ways listed in the table on page 48. Contrasting plus-points appear in the column to the right. Read through this list very carefully so you can recognize this mechanism at work in life and on the golf course. Use a dictionary if there is any doubt as to their meaning.

LIST OF COMMON OUT-POINTS AND
PLUS-POINTS AND THEIR DEFINITIONS

Out-Points	Plus-Points
Omitted data: failure to include information; to neglect; to fully observe. Resulting in: confusion.	All relevant facts known: see and know all relevant facts.
Altered importance: to modify the significance of information. Resulting in: never were sure of what you got in the first place.	Correct relative importance: found to be true as it relates to the solution.
Dropped out of time: to go out of present time. Resulting in: too much thinking inside the head.	Time properly noted: the moment of occurrence correctly observed.
False data: contrary to fact or truth; not true; incorrect. Resulting in: failure.	Data proven demonstrable: information shown true through experimentation.
Altered sequence of events: modification of logical order of items. Resulting in: loss of control.	Events in correct sequence: occurrences properly ordered in succession.
Data untrue unrelated: opposite information. Resulting in: too much significance.	Comparable data: information that can be regarded as similar.
Added inapplicable data: irrelevant, inappropriate, and unsuitable information joined to existing data. Resulting in: inconsistency.	Applicable data: information that can be applied.
Incorrectly included data: false information positioned in the correct place. Resulting in: thinking you're right when you're operating on false information.	Adequate data: barely satisfactory information; sufficient.
Wrong target: incorrect observation. Resulting in: miscalculations.	Correct target: accurate observation.
Wrong source: false opinion leaders. Resulting in: false data	Correct source: true opinion leader.
Falsehood: lack of accuracy or truth; a false belief or theory. Resulting in: ignorance.	Correct time, place, surroundings and event.
Contrary facts: opposite of what has been seen or is true. Resulting in: unable to confront true data.	Facts that bear out: what you observe.

In order to understand this mechanism and disarm it, you must take full responsibility for the errors or mistakes on the fairways or greens. You must fully understand the mechanics of out-points and plus-points (for example, hitting a green in regulation, making a birdie, making the right club selection). Assign responsibility to yourself for any and all mistakes—not the club, the ball, the course, the person next to you, or any of the other things that are readily available. It's you! You did it! If you can do this, you will be less prone to make mistakes and be fully able to apply your skills.

Golf is a game of blame or regret, responsibility versus accountability. With one, you're the loser; with the other, you're the winner. What can you do to take charge and handle the out-points? Next, we'll discuss the options.

THE MIND TRAP: PROBLEMS, SITUATIONS, AND SOLUTIONS

You have run into a problem on the golf course. Maybe it's your putting, your distance control, or something else that has gone astray. Well, your mind will solve this problem in one of the following ways:

1. Go after the problem with full force.

2. Pretend there is no problem.

3. Throw down your clubs and leave.

4. Do nothing about a known problem.

5. Give up the game of golf.

Now, let's apply these solutions. Let's say that you're faced with the following situation on the golf course: You're 150 yards out, and the flag is cut on the right edge of the green, guarded by water short and water right. You may decide to handle this in any of the following five ways.

1. **Your first option** is to go after the problem with full force. Champions become champions because they attack every situation they encounter with full force and don't waver from their goals. To become victorious, you must choose to stay on your intended course and attack your problems head-on. So go ahead and take direct aim at that flag and hit that ball!

2. **Your second option** is to pretend there is no problem here. You've heard this approach in flippant responses such as "I'm not worried," or "What water?" and the like. Thoughts like these get you further away from your attack mode, and you will surely hit the ball into the water.

3. **Your third option** is to throw down your clubs and leave. You'll take it up another day. Your inability to face up to the task takes over, and you start believing that you can't beat the problem, so you run away from it.

4. **Your fourth option** is to acknowledge the problem, but do nothing about it. You don't research the hole, test the grounds, and so forth. In this case, you know the water is to the right. There are things you can do, such as playing more to the left or safely long and left of the hole, instead you hit it to the right and smack dab into the water.

5. **Your fifth and worst option** available is to quit. This reflects an inability to confront and take responsibility for failure. The problem, which was set up to make the game interesting for the player, has now gotten the better of you, and you can't face it ever again. This is how someone quits. They have to be right about being wrong.

If you chose to deal with the problem head on—good! You have chosen correctly. But choosing to confront the problem does not mean looking into the mind for solutions. This is a tricky game. What you're trying to solve is not in your head. It is out on the golf course. Always look outward for your solutions. There is a whole world out there to help you solve your problems. You don't need thinking; you want knowingness.

Re-examine the five options above. They may help you choose the correct solution to the problem next time.

SO, WHERE DOES THE TROUBLE START?

It starts simply by thinking too much. If you take on a must-have attitude, you're just setting yourself up for a self-evaluation (described earlier). Psychologists tell us to think positive. Thinking is not *doing*. Thinking is inside your head. Golf is out on the course. There is no such thing as thinking positive. Doing positive is the only reality. Inside your head is a jungle. Outside is the world.

There is a huge difference between thinking and knowing. If you think positive, the only thing that will happen is you will think positive. But if you know with certainty, and you project that certainty into the future and hold it in place, your actions will head toward your knowingness.

When you hit a bad shot and are affected by it, you ponder it. This is self-evaluation. When you evaluate yourself, you are basically telling yourself that you are in a state of confusion. Your mind will then figure this and figure that, trying to come to some sort of solution. As we've said, evaluation is defined as the action of challenging your stable data without presenting new or better data to take the place of the challenged data. Evaluation leads to confusion.

Refuting and discrediting what you consider to be fact, to have demonstrated as skill, invalidates your knowingness. This causes doubt. Once you have mastered the basics of golf and are comfortable with them, never doubt yourself. Things will go wrong on the course mostly from misinformation you have processed in your mind and then apply on the course. A clear mind, with great perception and the ability to differentiate distance, speed, height, thrust, and curvature, is the route to a championship plan.

If you are a beginner or need help in improving your game, seek out a teacher who understands the differences between evaluation/invalidation and understanding/knowingness. Only through understanding and knowingness do you eliminate the noise and garble from the mind. A good teacher can deliver understanding and bypass the invalidation/evaluation mind scenario. They can deliver knowingness. Criticism never really helps anyone, but understanding can move mountains.

WHO'S REALLY PLAYING GOLF?

Who's playing anyway? Have you ever asked yourself this? Sometimes nothing goes right. Nothing you do seems to work. There is an explanation for this, and it's called Alternate Personality Syndrome. We talked about this earlier in the chapter, but we cannot understate the relevance of this to your golf game. It works like this:

The goal of the organism is to stay alive. The mind is set up to assure this goal is met. If you, the person, cannot deal with life or some crisis, then the mind will search its memory banks for some alternate solution based on a past viewpoint, acted out as an alternate personality who dealt with the crisis before and succeeded. That alternate could be in the form of a parent, sibling, or anyone else who has, in your viewpoint, survived or did better than you in a certain situation. The mind is always working and recording. It will search its memory banks and find this winning guy or gal and become them. Let's look at this again.

Remember, the mind has a hard time accepting failure. It's programmed to survive at any cost. It has been set up to protect and secure survival of the organism. If it cannot do that, it has to rationalize why this happened. It may also protect itself by assuming another identity. This identity is not capable of playing on the golf course. This is the main reason for frustration. You know you can make that shot, but you can't. Well, the truth is you can, but the alternate can't.

Look at this really closely. An announcer at some sporting event will comment on a player: "Well, if the real guy shows up today, he will be hard to beat" or, "Depending on who shows up, we might have a good game." They mean that some athletes, golfers, ballplayers, or sports figures are not consistent. They have moments of greatness but display mediocre play at other times. Why? It's because when the guy is good, it's *him.* When he is not, his alternate personality is running the show.

It all has to do with failure or nonsurvival. The alternate personalities—and there could be many—have been developed and manifested by the mind since childhood, only to be reactivated when you're under some great stress and can't face it. Someone has to step up and claim responsibility for the failure. More likely than not, it won't be you. It will be some alternate you. However, this alternate you doesn't have all your skills and talents. It tries to borrow some from you, but as we have seen on the playing field, the alternate-you athletes are not so good.

Alternate personalities can be contagious. One individual will suddenly turn around and become like another individual. We've seen this with whole teams or groups of people who assume one giant alter ego. An entire team may be infected, one player after another, until they're all in an altered state.

We've all heard golfers and ballplayers commenting about how they were just not themselves that day. Guess what? They weren't! We can fully dramatize a whole fake person or team and not even be aware of it. That's right. This alternate fake can't golf or do anything as good as the real person. But from the outside, people are observing the guy and commenting on how he's just not himself today.

This changeover might have taken place in a week, a day, or even moments before the event. Naturally, the best thing for the individual is to be his or her self. That's pretty hard to maintain. We've all complained from time to time that we're just not ourselves. But why does this happen? It happens when an invalidation or evaluation enters your mind from one or more directions or sources, such as self-to-self or another to you. You may hear others talking about your play, or you may tell another things like, "It looks like a tough course today" or "I hope I'm up to it." When self-doubt, confusion, invalidation, and evaluations are committed to you or by you, you open the door for these alternate personalities to step in and save you. These are mis-emotions and are caused by thinking too much. These transgressions against self, and even against others, invite all sorts of helpers to come in and justify your actions.

Human beings, despite all of their shortcomings, are basically good. When nonsurvival transgressions are committed against a fellow human being or self, the person needs to justify the action. Most of the time, the offender knows they did wrong and can't confront it, so they use an alternate self to explain it away. The only trouble is that once you call up this guy or gal, they stay around for a while being you. But they are not you, and they can't play golf.

Remember Sybil, the woman with the multiple personalities? To some degree, we all have multiple personalities lurking about that we put to use in different situations. For most of us, our minds keep things in order so that our everyday personality switches are barely perceptible. The mind uses many personalities to get through tough situations. You may have one personality at work, another for social events, and yet another when you play golf.

Everyone has those voices in their head. You can try to deny it, but you know they exist. Some of those voices are the voices of your alternate selves. Our goal is to keep those alternate voices under control in order to clear a path through the chaos of noise and confusion that can take you out of the game and out of present time. The techniques in the next chapter will show you how to do this.

But how? Simply keep the door closed to these alternate personalities by maintaining your integrity under *all* situations. Take full responsibility for any and all shortcomings or actions you may have committed, and remember, there are no real failures, only learning experiences. "Failure" is just another opportunity to observe and learn. You will then go from a state of not knowing to a state of knowingness. Never accept pity or sympathy, for this will freeze you in the past, trapped in a world of helpless confusion. Never allow evaluation or invalidation from others to infect you. You should give and seek only understanding about your game, and you will always be you. How refreshing is that? After all, who's better than you to play golf? No one!

Techniques to Eliminate Mind Noise

*I*n this chapter, you will find techniques for maintaining a balance of mind and ability by removing unwanted thoughts and voices in your head. These techniques are proven solutions to the problems stated previously in this book. For the first time in your life, take care, defeat the demons, and go free. Gain the ability to control life and livingness. Become the master of the golf ball, not its slave. The choice is yours.

THE BEGINNING OF THE JOURNEY

The search for silence within your mind and body will allow you to perform all tasks and skills at the ultimate level. It is a self-awakening. It is a journey into the self that will release you from the bonds of confusion and indecision. It is a vision that all is possible.

You must face the fact that you are a beginner in the sense that you have never been taught the real game of life. This information is probably new to you. A part of you has an urge to know it, to surpass yourself, for only those who realize the truth can perform at their optimum levels, only those who seek it can possibly even start to understand it.

WHAT YOU'RE UP AGAINST

There are basic steps of silencing that mind/body noise forever. But first you must face the total reality of your present-day condition. Here are the ABCs of life. Study them. Know them by heart. This is what you're up against.

A. You are not in control of your own thoughts.

B. You are not in control of your emotions.

C. You are a slave to a mind that thinks by reacting to stimulus from the environment.

D. You are imprisoned by unresolved past situations that affect the way you perceive things today.

E. Multiple personalities live within you, each one trying to be the leader.

F. Mis-emotion controls the hormones of your body, causing a negative effect.

G. Ego and having to be right lead to arguments within self.

H. Attachment and ownership are aberrations.

I. Your skills and abilities are performed at subpar levels and without consistency.

J. You lie to yourself every day.

K. You cannot confront certain things or people in life.

L. You do and think things that violate your integrity, morals, and ethical goals.

M. You do things to others that you wouldn't want done to you.

N. You allow things to happen that you wouldn't want happening to you.

O. You invalidate and evaluate.

P. You do not validate others' communications even if you disagree.

Q. You don't recognize the balance of force and intelligence.

R. You think and figure and agree with reality.

S. You don't know how to know. That education is not learning.

T. A lie will persist in your mind, but the truth will release you.

U. You don't disagree with the illusions of life. That what is, is not.

V. Life's barriers are necessary.

W. Time and space are an illusion.

X. You don't live in present time.

Y. You can become greater than you could ever imagine.

Z. Who you are is *you*, and what is—*is*.

Additional realities:

- Equality is a lie, and differentiation is the only truth.
- Stupidity stems from not looking, and not looking is the offspring of ego.

To have a full realization of who and what you are and clearly see your environment, it is necessary to fully understand yourself and the ABCs of an aberrant life. To do this, you must silence the aberrant noises in your head, destroying or changing them. The following techniques will do just that. Practice them and rise above your present self.

TECHNIQUES FOR SILENCING MIND NOISE

How do we obtain freedom from the voices and opinions within us? The road is clear. In order to do so, you must have the correct data to replace old ideas. Two objects cannot occupy the same space, so before new data can come in as fact, the old data must be removed. This is the law of affinity. You must get to know that data. You must believe in it and apply it. Then go out and play your game of golf. You will be so amazed at your abilities and skills that others will wonder what happened to you. Let them all wonder!

Let's look further. The mind of human beings has been a mystery! Generation after generation has sought this knowledge. Whole civilizations have disappeared for lack of understanding it.

From primitive man to present time, we have found ourselves in a state of helplessness, trying to understand this mystery. Why do we act and think and feel? Why is there aberration, illness, violence, sadness, and sorrow? In man's desperation to find the truth, he has drugged, melted, and removed the brains of many a poor sucker. It is in our view that, with the advent of psychiatry, we have driven people insane and broke. You cannot heal what you cannot find with modern psychiatry. The truth is never uncovered, only the illusions of truth. The aberration is occluded and hidden, otherwise it would not exist or persist. So how does one compose a solution to this monumental problem? We must look at what human beings try to do with thought and analyze how the mind influences that effort. What is the full potential of the mind, and what is its source of aberration? This is the basic view of what needs to be understood.

The optimum individual is one who has conquered the mind noise, thus eliminating the potential for illness and aberration. This person has increased their perception to see, hear, smell, taste, and touch. These are your lines to reality; these are your lines to any great skill, especially golf. How can you perceive reality if you do not possess 100 percent clarity of sense? How can you really see any golf course? How much do you really see, hear, touch, taste, and smell? How much do you really understand? How much of what you understand is aberration and how much is personality? What do you know of your past? What can you remember? Why is your past occluded? The mind has an ability to remember, why can't you? Why can't you remember how to hit that perfect drive?

Knowing and facing reality and confronting it are key aspects of mind silence. If you cannot perceive the past reality and confront it, then in a sense, you are not facing full reality, for reality is the connection of the past to the present to the future—it is one. You don't live as you were—you live as you're going to be. You live as you would in the future through imagination and cognition—envisioning future goals. This is the golf solution.

Rationalities are the products of perceiving, imagining, and solving problems using conclusions to solve further problems. This is the product of the silent mind. The fact of the matter is, a knowing being is incapable of error. The part of the mind that computes answers to problems deals in data only. It computes perfectly on the data stored and perceived. However, most of this is unreal data based on unreal solutions, unreal perceptions, and unreal realities. When incorrect data is taken into the mind, incorrect solutions come out. Essentially, the solution to aberrant mind noise and mis-emotion is to discover why the mind is subject to aberrant data. Why has the mind lost its ability to differentiate right from wrong? Why can't the mind sort out the correct solutions? Although human beings do evil, they are not evil. Quiet the aberrations, and the evil goes; and when it's gone, your life, your vigor, and your personality soar! You'll act—not react. You will have determination of self. You can choose. You are confident. You then can live and play any game you choose—especially golf.

The following exercises will help to calm the mind. Begin by setting aside a few minutes of quiet time for yourself each day. Try to do this exercise at roughly the same time. Dedicate this time to yourself.

PROCEDURE ONE Focusing Your Concentration

Start by choosing an object to concentrate on that you can hold in your hand. Let's use a golf ball. Sit down in a comfortable chair in a dimly lit room that is free from distractions. Hold the golf ball about arm's length in front of you at eye level and concentrate on it and nothing else. Time yourself to see how long it takes for thoughts to enter your mind.

No doubt, it won't take long. At this point a very interesting thing will occur to you. You will realize that, unfortunately, you have little or no control over your own thoughts. It will be frustrating at first and a little frightening to really understand that you are not in control of your own thoughts. That you are a slave to all that mish-mash you call thinking, and that the body you're in could care less about you and will act as it pleases according to some program you have *no* say over.

As you practice each day, try to lengthen the duration of time you can go without thoughts intruding. Today you may be a beginner in this new world, but don't despair. In time, those uncontrolled thoughts and urges will disappear, or at least lessen in intensity. You should be able to do this at will and for as long as you want. That is control. That is the goal.

PROCEDURE TWO   Quieting the Mind

After you have mastered concentration, the next best thing is for you to start quieting your mind. Sit quietly, undisturbed, in a pleasant place. Close your eyes halfway and go deep into your consciousness. Unlike the previous exercise, this exercise does not focus your concentration on an object. Removing the object makes it much more difficult to keep intrusions out. Be very careful to keep your mind's door bolted shut. Beware, unpleasant thoughts will enter on the back of pleasant thoughts like thieves and create confusion. If you commit yourself to this process, and do it regularly, you will eventually become strong enough so that even mis-emotion and destructive thoughts will be easily transformed or rejected. This is the beginning of your freedom from slavery.

Eventually, you will have to confront and accept the challenge and conquer these wrong thoughts leading to mis-emotions, for the world is made up of these and they will always be present. It is your duty to transform these mis-thoughts and mis-emotions, but only when you are in a position to do so safely. Do this exercise once a day for as long as it takes until you can attain at least fifteen to twenty minutes of a quieted mind. Once you have mastered it, you own it forever, and you no longer need to practice it.

PROCEDURE THREE   Silencing the Mind

Let's start with the basics. Find a corner of your room, a place of quiet, peaceful surroundings. It is advisable to wear clean, light colored or white garments. Colors have a wavelength to them that affects the mind. Each exercise builds upon the previous in difficulty. At this point, we require light colored or white garments. It is important to keep the body relaxed and comfortable. Proper breathing is very important. Try to breathe in as slowly and quietly as possible. Leave a short pause between exhaling and inhaling.

With every inhale, bring calmness into the body. With every exhale, push out mis-emotions like fear, anger, anxiety, ego, and attachment. Feel that you are breathing out all the rubbish inside you. Breathe out the mis-emotions—anything inside you that you recall or recognize from the ABCs list on page 56—anything that you no longer want to claim as your own.

If you practice this method of breathing, you will soon feel its results. If you can breathe this way for five minutes every day, you will be able to make fast progress. The breathing must be done in a very conscious way—not mechanically. As you reach an advanced stage of breathing, you can feel the negative energy as it is released: internally, from your limbs, your head, your skin, through every part of your body. This can and will happen very quickly. As you do this, you should feel the restlessness leaving and, with this, the noise in your head quieting down. There are seven trillion cells in the body. Each one has its say. That's a lot of noise. As you breathe, you should feel there is not a single place in your body that is not being occupied by the flow of that breath.

Keep your eyes slightly open while doing this, for it is very easy to fall into a dream world if they are closed. There is no dynamic energy in this state, only lethargy and self-complacency. You must remain alert and on a mission to rid your inner self of its aberrant noises. Concentrate on your breathing with your eyes half open and half closed. And while you're going deep within, focus your conscious attention both on the inner and outer worlds. At some point, you will experience a "separateness" from your body. You will have a cognition that you are not your body, but just you—a separate entity, operating within a body and using it to contact the environment.

The outer world with its distractions, the inner world with its noise, and the dreamy world of sleep will all be inviting. But you must fight their allure. You are challenging these worlds and making a statement of victory that you are alert and these worlds cannot control you. Remember, your eyes should remain slightly open. It will help you remember that you belong to this world. You are maintaining control over the voices and noise in your head. The moment any unwanted noise, negative thought, or mis-emotion enters your mind, cut it to pieces. Soon you will be able to not only conquer this inner world, but the outside world. The world will be yours to conquer.

Just remember, your life grows weaker the moment your mind becomes prey to self-indulgent thoughts. Cut off bad thoughts and kill them. How do you do this? Just bring that thought or urge or mis-emotion right in front of you the moment you recognize it for what it is, and it will disappear. If at first you don't have the capacity to do this, don't despair. Just don't give that thought any more importance. Treat it as insignificant, and don't give it any energy or validation. The more you practice, the more power you will gain. It will come to you. There are no setbacks or losses here, only abilities gained. If you cannot at first handle these thoughts, it is not a loss, it is a win. For the first time in your life, you have served notice that you are coming and will continue to be in control.

TECHNIQUES FOR BEING HERE NOW

The purpose of the following exercises is to help you increase your ability to remain in the here and now and to further conquer the voices of doom in your mind that prevent you from getting up to the speed of life and playing your best.

PROCEDURE ONE Present Time Here and Now

In order to be free from past transgressions, enjoy happiness, experience superior intelligence, and overcome obstacles toward your goals, complete this procedure. Remember, transgressions are the single source of misfortune and illness. All aberrations and irrational behaviors are caused by the restimulation of past transgressions. They are stimulus/mind responses and are antisurvival.

Find a quiet place to sit. Have a pen and paper with you. Make sure you will not be disturbed. You are going to search your mind for any present or past transgressions. At first it may be difficult to confront them, and they will try to hide from your viewing, but if you are truly willing to help yourself, they will appear. Just keep at it. It's worth it!

Once you become conscious of a transgression, write it up as outlined below.

Step One: State the transgression.

Example: I stole an apple from a grocery store when no one was looking.

Step Two: Write up the event addressing who, where, when, how, and why.

Example: Who: *Me, myself*

Where: *The corner grocery on Fifth and Lane. The apples were outside on a stand.*

When: *It was noon in August.*

How: *I looked around and didn't see anyone, so I quickly took the apple and put it in my pocket.*

Why: *I was hungry. I figured I could get away with it, I could save a quarter. Why not?*

Step Three: Cognition.

Example: I realize it was not okay to take what does not belong to me. I wouldn't want it to happen to me, and I did cause someone else a loss.

The recognition of each transgression will release the negative energy from your mind and leave only a memory. The more transgressions you become aware of, the freer your mind will become. This process could take anywhere from a week to a month to finish. See it to the end and you will profoundly raise your awareness of life. This new awareness can only be a boom to your golf pursuits.

PROCEDURE TWO   In the Moment

This next exercise will help ground you in the moment. Whether you're at home or on the golf course, find a quiet place—perhaps under a shady tree—sit down, get comfortable, and close your eyes.

Now visualize a golf ball just two feet to the left of you. Hold that vision in your mind.

Next, place another golf ball two feet to the right of you. Hold these two positions steady in your mind.

Now, place another golf ball two feet above your head. While holding these three positions steady, visualize holding a golf ball two feet below you.

Then place another ball two feet in back of you.

Finally, while holding all five golf balls still, place another golf ball two feet in front of you. Hold all six golf balls steady in your mind, visualizing all six positions.

Do this procedure until you have successfully mocked up all six balls and held them steadily in place without their moving or disappearing, or having any other thought come into your head. This works by giving the mind the ability to hold all points in the environment around you without any noise or any other consideration. This kind of absolute concentration will allow you to remain in the here and now while playing golf.

PROCEDURE THREE Extraction from Looking Within

Not being present in present time is actually being elsewhere. Usually, this "elsewhereness" occurs when you get stuck thinking about a past moment or past moments. In golf, this frequently happens when you suddenly hit a bad shot. You find yourself stuck in your head, repeating the incident. You can get pulled out of present time and back into your head thinking and remembering how bad the shot was or the consequences attached to that shot. You can see how subtly this mechanism can trap someone in their head, providing the perfect recipe for distracting attention from the task at hand—their next shot!

The following procedure will stop you from thinking, remembering, or attempting to correct a mistake by looking for some answer in your head. Remember, the answer is not in your head. The ability to perform the task is already programmed in your mind as your talent—your skill. Looking for a solution to something you already know how to do will cause your mind to freeze up by pitting confusion against solution.

To stop you from looking within, this next procedure asks you to look at objects in order to take your attention to an exterior object in present time. Next time you find yourself elsewhere on the golf course, do the following procedure by looking and locating things.

1. Locate the flagstick.

2. Locate your golf ball.

3. Locate your golf bag.

4. Locate the green.

5. Locate a tree.

6. Locate the tee box area.

7. Locate another person.

Repeat this procedure until you feel you are firmly rooted in your surroundings and less stuck in your head.

IN CONCLUSION

Well, it has been a long—and we're sure—revealing journey into the inner workings of the human mind. We hope that we have shed a little light on the golfer's dilemma of why "Sometimes I can" and "Sometimes I can't." If you look closely at sport statistics, you'll realize that a .300 batting average in baseball represents a player who is performing at less than one-third of their ability, and a golf score of sixty-two is far from a perfect score of eighteen. Some would say it is statistically impossible to shoot an eighteen in golf. But if your game was only at 50 percent, you would still be shooting a score of thirty-six. Most of us haven't even come close to reaching our real potential. Human beings have managed to trap themselves in their own prison of stupidity and apathy, but there is help.

Every problem has a solution, and it is within the problem itself that the answer may be found. Keep emotions at bay, and stay calm. Assemble all the facts without bias or rumor. Lay out all the component parts of a problem. Never use reckless force. Spiritual understanding will inevitably produce the best possible solution. Get wise council, but don't ever forget that human beings have been blessed with intuition—follow it, and don't forget that the opposite of intuition is emotion. If you shut down your stimulus/emotion-driven mind, and let yourself drift into an analytical state, you will produce the answers you're looking for.

As in life, so goes golf, a tough but conquerable game. You can be its master. You can rule the fairways. All you have to do is believe.

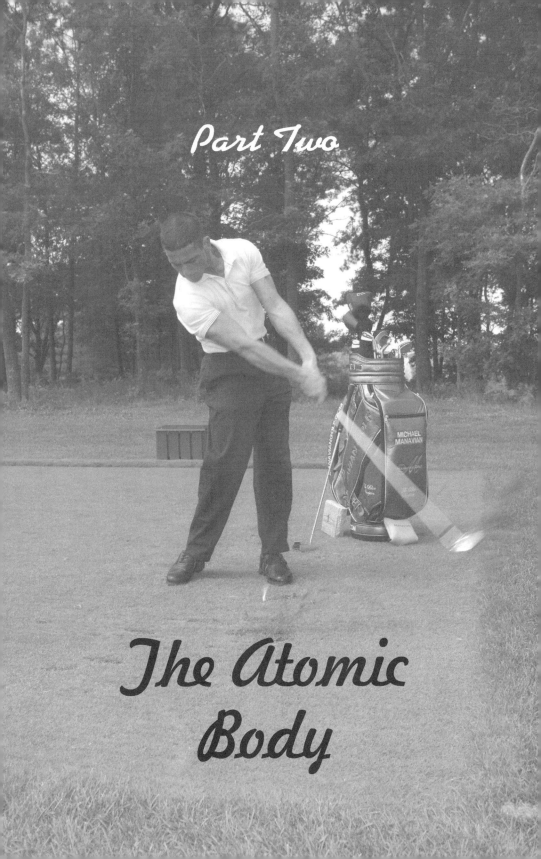

Part Two

The Atomic
Body

7

Anatomy, Physiology, and the Training Effect

To fully understand and master golf, it is important to understand how the body works. Similar to owning a car, it helps to understand what this large, powerful machine is. The machine you employ in life, and certainly in golf, is the human body. While the mind runs this incredible machine, the body delivers the action in the game. Yet most golfers are oblivious to the significant role the body plays in the game of golf.

The human body is a biomechanical machine that requires maintenance and upgrading. Unfortunately, although it is critical to understand how the body responds to training and conditioning, the human body does not come with an owner's manual. So how do you maintain your body and keep it performing at peak

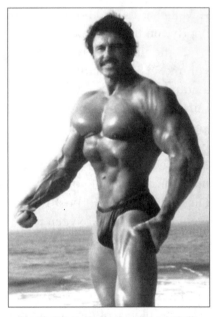

Mr. Universe's body was a totally built machine.

levels when you know little about its main components?

In this chapter we will provide you with valuable information regarding the main strategies for achieving and maintaining a well-conditioned body. Brief and to the point, it will supply you with insights into how and why the body responds to highly intense exercise, as well as the role each system and part plays in the quest for fitness. Knowledge is power. Harness this power, and you will reap the benefits on and off the golf course.

LUNGS

Air consists of 21 percent oxygen and 79 percent nitrogen, and the volume of air you can process (bring in and push out) is the first limiting factor in exercise. Lungs have no muscles of their own. They depend completely on the rib cage and diaphragm muscles. The stronger these muscles are, the greater the capacity of the lungs to consume oxygen.

Vital capacity refers to how much of the actual lungs can be brought into action, or simply, the amount of air you can exhale after a deep breath. A well-conditioned body will utilize much more of its lung capacity than a poorly conditioned body.

Some air always remains in the lungs. This air is referred to as residual volume. It is difficult to exhale too much of the residual volume. The amount remaining in the lungs limits the amount of air you can breathe in, causing shortness of breath. A large volume of residual air in the lungs prevents that portion of the lungs from working properly. If you allow your body to deteriorate, the usable portion of your lungs will be limited. No matter how nutritionally sound you are, you can only physically perform up to the capacity of your lungs. Strong and powerful lungs enable anyone, including golfers, to breathe in without effort, thus allowing life-giving, thought-processing oxygen to enter the brain.

BLOOD

The bloodstream is the body's assembly line. Red blood cells are the carriers in the blood, filling up and emptying their contents then returning for a refill. Hemoglobin in the red cells carries oxygen. The number of red blood cells available determines the body's vitality. Exercise increases the number of red blood cells, thus more hemoglobin, which in turn produces more oxygen and more vitality. It stands to reason that a well-conditioned body will have a greater volume of blood to work with, thereby enriching all the cells and removing their waste products.

Exercise is responsible for the development of new vascular passageways, which aid in endurance and fatigue-fighting factors. Exercise increases the size of the blood vessels, allowing for unrestricted flow and helping control blood pressure.

CELLS AND TISSUE

Cells are the basic structure and functional units of an organism. There are many types of cells in the body, each differentiated by their task. Among the many kinds of cells are muscle and blood cells. Each cell is like a small factory with receiving and shipping storerooms and power plants. These factories require nutrients and oxygen to run.

The next higher level of structure in the body is tissue. Tissue is made up from groups of cells that perform special functions. Exercise fires up the cells and tissues, keeping them rich with blood, nutrients, and oxygen. Exercise keeps cells and tissues healthy and in repair. If you don't use your body, it will start deteriorating at the cellular level. Premature aging of bones and muscles is a direct condition of lack of cellular action brought about by poor circulation of blood, nutrition, and oxygen. Exercise stimulates, refreshes, and rejuvenates these tissues.

ORGANS OF DIGESTION

Different kinds of tissues are joined to form an even higher level of organization called organs. There are many different organs of structure and function. You don't need to be knowledgeable about them all—only the ones that will aid in your understanding of exercise conditioning and emotion.

Stomach

The stomach is a J-shaped enlargement of the gastrointestinal tract located directly under the diaphragm in the left region of the abdomen. The inlet is the esophagus; the outlet is the intestines. When empty, the stomach is about the size of a sausage; however, when full, it can stretch to an incredible size. The passage of solid food or semisolid food from mouth to stomach takes approximately four to eight seconds. Soft foods and liquids take only a second.

The stomach mixes the food into a sort of pulp, using a wave motion. The primary chemical activity of the stomach is to begin the digestion of protein through the use of the enzyme pepsin. Pepsin can only operate in an acidic base. It becomes inactive in an alkaline environment. Protein promotes an acid base. Starch and carbohydrates promote an alkaline base. (Fat digestion relies almost exclusively on enzymes found in the small intestine.)

The stomach empties all of its contents two to six hours after ingestion. Foods rich in carbohydrates leave the stomach in a few hours. Proteins are somewhat slower. The process is slowest after fats have been consumed. All kinds of athletes, from golfers to marathon runners to weightlifters, perform at their best on an empty stomach, after all digestion is completed and the blood has delivered the nutrients to their respective destinations. Muscles rich with blood, oxygen, and nutrients will perform at their absolute peak. Food that is undigested or going through the digestive process will rob the cells of their vitality because the blood is being used in the digestive tract. The digestive process requires a great deal of energy from start to finish. To exercise while this process is taking place cannot serve you very well.

Intestines

The intestines are the long, tubelike portion of the gastrointestinal tract extending from the stomach to the anus and completing the process of digestion. It consists of the small and large intestines. Most food absorption takes place in the small intestine, where food travels after the stomach. Digestion is aided by the pancreas, liver, and gallbladder, which together produce enzymes and other fluids used during digestion and absorption. After most of the nutrients have been extracted in the small intestine, the resulting slurry goes to the large intestine. There, excess water is removed and the waste is prepared for evacuation.

Pancreas

The pancreas is a spongy, six-inch-long gland made up of clusters of cells. It is connected to the small intestines by a series of ducts. One percent of these cells form the endocrine portion of the pancreas, secreting the hormones glucagon, insulin, and somatostatin. The remaining 99 percent of cells release a mixture of digestive enzymes designed to digest specific foods.

Liver

The liver is the largest organ in the body. Located under the diaphragm and occupying most of the right portion of the abdomen, the liver weighs about three and a half pounds and measures about eight inches across by six and a half inches down. Like the pancreas, it is connected to the small intestine by a series of ducts.

The liver is divided into right and left lobes, which are separated by a ligament. The lobes of the liver are made up of functional units. These units destroy worn out white and red blood cells and bacteria, as well as remove toxins from the blood. Poisons are stored or detoxified. Products made by the liver and nutrients needed by other cells are secreted back into the blood.

This organ performs many vital functions:

- It manufactures and secretes bile, which is used in the small intestine for the emulsification and absorption of fats. It is impossible to lose body fat if the liver is overworked or not functioning to its capacity.

- It produces albumin, which is the main protein component of blood.

- It destroys worn out red and white blood cells and some bacteria.

- It contains enzymes that either break down or transform toxic biochemical products produced by the body into less harmful compounds. When amino acids are burned for energy, for example, they leave behind toxic nitrogenous wastes, such as ammonia, that are converted to urea by the liver cells. Moderate amounts of urea are harmless to the body and are easily excreted by the kidneys and sweat glands.

- It is involved in carbohydrate metabolism, either storing or releasing glucose, depending on the body's energy needs.

- It stores glycogen, copper, iron, and the fat-soluble vitamins A, D, E, and K, as well as some toxins that cannot be broken down and excreted. (High levels of DDT are found in the livers of animals, including humans, who eat sprayed fruits and vegetables.)

- Along with the kidneys, it participates in the activation of vitamin D.

Kidneys

The kidneys are a pair of reddish bean-shaped organs found just above the waist near the posterior wall of the abdomen. They monitor the blood for waste products, help regulate the body's natural balance of nutrients and amino acids, and produce urine.

The metabolism of nutrients results in the production of wastes by body cells, including carbon dioxide and excess water. Catabolism (the breakdown of molecules for energy) produces toxic wastes such as carbon dioxide, lactic acid, ammonia, and urea.

The primary function of the urinary system, and therefore the kidneys, is to help keep the body in homeostasis (a state of equilibrium between the interrelated functions and elements of the body) by controlling the composition and volume of the blood. It does so by removing and restoring selected amounts of water and dissolved substances. The kidneys regulate the composition and volume of the blood and remove wastes from the blood in the form of urine. They excrete selected amounts of various wastes, help control blood pH, and help regulate blood pressure.

As the kidneys go about their activities, they remove many materials from the blood, return the ones that the body requires, and eliminate the remainder. The eliminated materials are collectively called urine. The entire volume of blood in the body is filtered by the kidneys approximately sixty times a day.

HEART

The heart is the center of the cardiovascular system. It is a hollow, muscular organ that weighs about eleven ounces and beats more than one hundred thousand times a day to pump blood through more than sixty thousand miles of blood vessels. The blood vessels form a network of tubes that carry blood from the heart to the tissues of the body and then return it to the heart.

The heart is situated obliquely between the lungs. It is shaped like a blunt cone that's about the size of your closed fist. This is the magnificent engine that keeps the whole assembly line going. It takes oxygen-laden blood from the lungs and pumps it throughout the body, while taking carbon dioxide–laden blood from the body and pumping it into the lungs, where it is exchanged for more oxygen.

The heart began its work before you were born. It is working now, and will continue to work your entire life. Ironically, the heart works less efficiently when you give it little to do than it does when you make it work more. Obesity, stress, and many other factors can, of course, speed up your heart rate considerably, even though you may appear to be in great condition. Even at complete rest, an unconditioned person who does not exercise forces their heart to beat nearly thirty thousand times more each day of their life. An unconditioned heart beats harder and less efficiently than a conditioned heart performing the same activity.

The heart tissue is all muscle. Unlike the lungs, the heart does its own work—without doubt the most important work in the body. The health of its tissue depends on its size and how well it is supplied with blood vessels. An athlete's heart is strong and healthy. It is relatively large and highly efficient, pumping more blood with less effort. Like any well-conditioned athlete, it accomplishes great things seemingly effortlessly.

The health of the heart is dependent on several factors. First and foremost, a healthy heart depends on the health of its tissue, and healthy cardiac tissue depends on its saturation from large, healthy, arteries. For its own energy requirements, the heart needs the same supply of oxygen that it pumps to the other tissues in the body. This saturation coverage, or vascularizaton, is one of the most important benefits of the training effect and is nowhere more evident or more important than it is in the heart.

The second factor that indicates the health of the heart is the heart rate. Conditioned hearts, as they grow larger and stronger, can beat more slowly because they're pumping more blood with each stroke. Exercise reduces maximum heart rates, which is important. Healthy hearts will peak, without strain, at 190 beats per minute or less, while poorly conditioned hearts may go as high as 220 beats or more during exhausting activity. This is dangerously high. Exercise conditions the heart by strengthening it so that it can hold near-maximum rates for longer periods before fatigue sets in.

Another factor that affects heart rate is called the anticipatory rate, or tension rate. You might think of it as the emotional heart rate. The heart's ability to respond to mental, as well as physical, stimuli make it a unique muscle. Crisis affects the heart rate, but training can reduce this effect.

Two systems in your body prepare you for "fight or flight" response by increasing the heart rate to rush in more oxygen before you've even made a move. In periods of acute emotional stress, the nervous system speeds up most of the body's activities and combines with the adrenal glands to produce a high level of hormones in the blood. When these hormones reach the heart, they cause an increase in the rate and strength of contraction.

A deconditioned heart does not always have the ability to slow down after a sudden stimulus. The heart may keep beating at an excessively fast rate, which could lead to a heart attack. With a conditioned heart, there's a better balance. After experiencing a sudden stimulus, you can still maintain control and never reach a high, potentially damaging level of hormones.

This, too, is part of the training effect. Either because of decreased production or more efficient utilization of hormones, a conditioned body is not as affected by excess hormones. Add to this the fact that a conditioned heart is already trained to level off at a relatively low maximum rate and you have built-in protection against uncontrollable emotional crisis. A deconditioned body doesn't have this protection. If a person also tends to be hyper-reactive (someone who gets overly excited, even in minor emergencies), then that person has two strikes against them—too much emotion and too little built-in physical protection.

The training effect benefits the heart in several ways by developing a strong, healthy muscle that works more effortlessly during moments of realization or moments of peak physical exertion. By doing so, the heart maintains large reserves of power to handle whatever physical or emotional stress is imposed upon it.

SLEEP

Human beings need sleep. We sleep and awaken in a fairly constant twenty-four-hour cycle. Just as there are different levels of consciousness, there are different levels of sleep. Normal sleep consists of two levels: non-rapid eye movement (non-REM), and rapid eye movement (REM). About 75 percent of total sleep time in adults is non-REM sleep. This is divided into the following four stages:

- **Stage 1:** The person is relaxing with eyes closed. During this time, respirations are regular, pulse is even, and the person has fleeting thoughts. If awakened, the person will frequently claim they had not been sleeping.

- **Stage 2:** It is harder to awaken the person. Fragments of dreams may be experienced, and the eyes may slowly roll from side to side.

- **Stage 3:** The person is very relaxed. Body temperature begins to fall and blood pressure decreases. It is difficult to wake the person. This stage occurs about twenty minutes after falling asleep.

- **Stage 4:** Deep sleep occurs. The person is very relaxed and responds slowly if awakened. This is the stage where most dreaming occurs.

Approximately ninety minutes into this deep REM sleep, human growth hormone, also known as somatotropin, is released. Somatotropin's function is to turn on the growth of body cells. It acts on the skeleton and skeletal muscles, in particular, to increase their rate of growth and maintain their size and strength. It does this by increasing the rate at which protein enters the cells. Growth hormone also promotes fat burning by commanding the cells to use fat as energy, and it stimulates cells to release fat to be burned by body cells.

It is obvious how important sleep becomes once a person decides to take on an exercise regimen. It is important to eat protein approximately one and a half to two hours before bedtime and to maintain absolute abstinence from carbohydrates three hours prior to sleep. Sugars and carbohydrates restrict the function of human growth hormone. You only grow when you sleep, so keep good sleep habits.

EXERCISE IS NECESSARY

We hope this brief journey into the workings of the body will help you understand the necessity of exercise. The next chapter delves deeper into the importance of proper nutrition and eating correctly and its role in helping to maintain a high level of conditioning. Now, let's continue our journey.

8

Nutrition and Diet

If you want to be successful at golf, you need to provide your body with everything it needs. Just as gas is to an engine, food is to the human body, and just as people value gold, diamonds, and precious jewels, the human body values nutrient-rich foods. Food is the body's prime source of fuel, and it is needed to meet both the body's energy needs and nutritional requirements. In order to improve your physical performance and to play to your full potential, you need to understand the basics of nutrition.

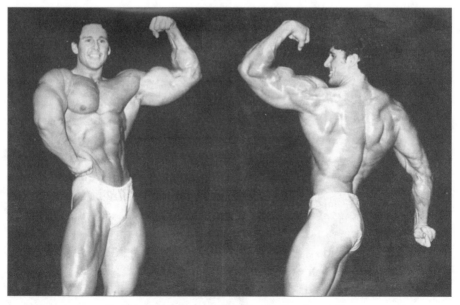

Optimal nutrition produces optimal results.

METABOLISM

Nutrients are chemical substances in food that provide energy, form new body components, or assist in the functioning of various body processes. There are six principal classes of nutrients: carbohydrates, proteins, lipids (fats), vitamins, minerals, and water. Carbohydrates, proteins, and fats (lipids) are digested by enzymes in the gastrointestinal tract. The end products of digestion are different forms of sugar, amino acids, and fatty acids. Some of these nutrients are used to manufacture new structural molecules or to synthesize new regulatory molecules, such as hormones and other enzymes. Most nutrients, however, are used to produce energy to sustain life processes involving active transport, DNA replication, synthesis of proteins and other molecules, muscle contraction, nerve-impulse control, and other basic functions.

Some minerals and many vitamins are essential to the enzyme systems. They catalyze the reactions involved in the breakdown of carbohydrates, proteins, and lipids so they can become useful to the body. And water is responsible for and involved in nearly every bodily process.

Metabolism refers to all the chemical reactions of the body. The body's metabolism may be thought of as an energy-balancing act between catabolic (breaking down) reactions, which provide energy, and anabolic reactions (building up), which require energy.

Catabolism is the term for decompositional chemical reactions that provide energy. Digestion is a catabolic process in which the breaking down of food molecules into smaller molecules releases energy. Oxidation, also a catabolic process, is the removal of electrons and hydrogen from a molecule, or, less commonly, the addition of oxygen to a molecule. Glucose (sugar) is the body's favorite nutrient for oxidation, but fats and proteins are also oxidized. As substances are oxidized, energy is produced.

The opposite of catabolism is anabolism. Anabolism is a series of synthetic reactions whereby small molecules are built up into the larger ones that form the body's structural and functional components. Anabolic reactions require energy, which is provided by the body's catabolic reactions. Fats also participate in the body's anabolism. For instance, fats can be built into the phospholipids that form the plasma membrane. They also form the basis of the steroid hormones.

When the body needs energy, the glycogen stored in the liver is broken down into glucose and released into the bloodstream to be transported to cells, where it will be catabolized. This process, called glycogenolysis, usually occurs between meals.

As mentioned, there are six major nutrients essential to a well-conditioned body. A deficiency in only one of these major nutrients can leave you performing at less than your full potential, or even cause harm to your health.

CARBOHYDRATES

These macronutrients are the main source of instantly available energy for all your activities—both internal and external. There are basically two types of carbohydrates: simple (fast-acting) and complex (slow-acting). Simple carbohydrates include sugars, starches, and refined processed foods. Complex carbohydrates include vegetables (preferably green), fruits, seeds and nuts, and whole grains and their products.

How fast the body's supply of energy is depleted depends on the type of carbohydrate consumed because of the steps involved in storing the carbohydrate and transforming it into glucose, which is the body's preferred form of carbohydrate fuel. Refined carbohydrates are depleted quickly, while more complex carbohydrates are used up more slowly. During the process of digestion, polysaccharides and disaccharides (complex carbohydrates) are hydrolyzed to become monosaccharides (simple carbohydrates)—glucose, fructose, and galactose. They are then carried to the liver, where fructose and galactose are converted to glucose (sugar). The liver is the only organ that has the necessary enzymes to make this conversion. Thus, the story of carbohydrate metabolism is really the story of glucose metabolism.

If glucose is not needed immediately for energy, it is combined with many other molecules of glucose to form a long chain molecule called glycogen. This process, mediated by insulin in response to high glucose levels, is called glycogenesis. The body can store about 500 grams of glycogen in the liver and cells of the skeletal muscle. Roughly 80 percent of the glycogen is stored in the skeletal muscle.

Since glucose is the body's preferred source of energy, the fate of absorbed glucose depends on the energy needs of the body's cells. If the cells require immediate energy, the glucose is oxidized by the cells and converted to adenosine triphosphate (ATP), which is the main intracellular energy source. The glucose not needed for immediate use is handled in several ways. First, the liver can convert excess glucose to glycogen. Second, if the glycogen storage areas are filled up, the liver cells can transform the glucose to fat that can be stored in adipose tissue. Later, when the cells need energy, the glycogen and fat can be converted back to glucose, which is released into the bloodstream so it can be transported to cells for oxidation. Without the inhibiting effects of fats, the stomach empties its contents quickly, and the carbohydrates are digested at the same time.

FATS (LIPIDS)

And then there's fat. In general, people don't consider fats to be an important macronutrient in their diet. Fats have gotten much bad press, but they do serve a purpose. Fats work with vitamins to assure their absorption. They are a secondary form of energy after carbohydrates, and they help manufacture hormones and enhance their performance.

There are basically three kinds of fats: unsaturated, hydrogenated, and saturated. Unsaturated fats are good fats. They contain essential fatty acids, which are necessary for your growth and the prevention of heart disease. Hydrogenated fats, also called trans-fatty acids, are not good. They are made solid by the addition of the chemical hydrogen (a process known as hydrogenation) and act in destructive ways. Read labels! Saturated fats are found primarily in animal products such as fatty meats like beef, veal, and lamb, cheese, butter, and lard. They contain an unusual amount of carbon molecules within the fatty acids, which makes them difficult for the body to digest, but easy to store.

Oxidized fatty acids and high levels of "bad" cholesterol lead to cardiovascular disease. This happens because these fatty cells can penetrate artery walls, setting off an inflammatory reaction that injuries the artery and forms plaque deposits. A class of nutrients called antioxidants can help reduce these oxidative reactions by protecting cells against attack from oxidized cholesterol and fatty acids. Taking a quality antioxidant can go a long way in preventing cellular damage. A good health food store will contain many good antioxidant products.

While certain unsaturated fats such as certain vegetable oils (e.g., canola oil, olive oil, safflower oil and sunflower oil) and fish oils are important to include in a healthy diet, bad fats can negatively affect the efficiency of your body. The body will run at less than peak levels and compromise your skills. If you let this continue without intelligent intervention, you're playing Russian roulette with your life. There are many wonderful fat and butter substitutes on the market today—again, read labels.

Lipids such as fatty acids may oxidize to produce cellular energy, similar to carbohydrates. Each gram of fat produces about 9 calories. If the body has no immediate need to utilize fats, they are stored in the skin as adipose tissue (fat depots), throughout the body and in the liver.

The major function of adipose tissue is to provide storage for fats until they are needed for energy in other parts of the body. It also insulates and protects. About 50 percent of stored fat is deposited in subcutaneous tissue and 5 to 8 percent between the muscles. Fats are renewed approximately once every two to three weeks. Therefore, the fat stored in your adipose tissue today is not the same fat that was there last month. Fat is continually released from storage, transported, and redeposited into adipose tissue cells.

The body can store much more fat than it can glycogen. Moreover, the energy yield of fats is more than twice that of carbohydrates. Fats are the body's second favorite source of energy. But before fat molecules can be metabolized as an energy source, they must first be released from fat depots, a process that is stimulated by growth hormone.

Liver cells burn fat, carbohydrates, and protein. When a greater amount of carbohydrates enters the body than is needed for energy, or that can be stored as glycogen, the carbohydrates will be manufactured into fats in a process enhanced by insulin. This process is called lipogenesis. This holds true for amino acids as well. When people have more proteins in their diet than can be utilized, much of the excess protein is converted to, and stored as, fat.

PROTEIN

Proteins are involved in nearly every cell in the body. They serve as enzymes, cell transporters, and building blocks for muscle and skeletal tissue. Protein itself is made up of its own building blocks called amino acids. There are twenty standard amino acids, of which nine are essential. The body uses these nine amino acids to make the other eleven it needs. A protein food is called complete if it contains these nine essential acids; it's called incomplete if it's missing any one of the nine, thus rendering it useless. When someone eats a diet lacking in these nine essential amino acids, they go into a protein deficit, which will cause weakness, low energy, and mental and emotional problems. The body becomes more receptive to infection, wounds heal slowly, and muscles and bones are constantly sore. Foods such as beans, grains, soy products, tofu, and lentils are essentially ineffective because they are incomplete proteins. Foods such as dairy products, meats, and fish are complete proteins and perform all the tasks assigned to them.

Amino acids enter body cells by active transport. This process is stimulated by growth hormone. Almost immediately after entrance, they are synthesized into proteins. Generally, the body uses very little protein for energy, as long as it ingests or stores sufficient amounts of carbohydrates and fats. Each gram of protein produces about 4 calories.

During the process of digestion, proteins are broken down into their constituent amino acids. The amino acids are then absorbed by the blood capillaries through the villi, and transported to the liver via the hepatic portal vein. A certain amount of protein catabolism occurs in the body each day. Proteins are extracted from worn-out cells and broken down, making new proteins. If other energy sources are used up, the liver can convert protein to fat or glucose (sugar), or oxidize it to carbon dioxide and water.

Protein anabolism involves the formation of new proteins. Protein synthesis is stimulated by growth hormone, thyroxin, and insulin. Because protein is a primary ingredient of most cell structures, including muscle tissue, high-protein diets are essential during exercise.

Of the amino acids (protein building-blocks) needed by the body, nine are considered essential amino acids. These amino acids cannot be synthesized by the human body from molecules present in the body; they must be consumed in food (more on this later).

When your liver runs low on glycogen, and you do not eat foods containing these essential amino acids, your body starts catabolizing proteins. However, unless you are starving, large-scale fat and protein catabolism does not happen. Both fat molecules and protein molecules may be converted in the liver to glucose. Low-calorie diets insufficient to energy needs can bring about this catabolizing, or wasting away.

VITAMINS

Everyone needs vitamins. Any type of athlete needs more vitamins than most other people. Each vitamin has specific responsibilities in your body. For example, vitamin C is an important antioxidant that is involved in the production of essential enzymes; the B vitamins are essential for the con-version of energy; and vitamin E is an important antioxidant that is also involved in immune system support and DNA repair.

It is well established that athletes need an abundance of vitamins for optimal performance. Training uses up these substances, making it more critical that they be replenished. In the interest of "insurance," it's probably wise to take a quality natural (not synthetic) multivitamin from a reputable source at least once a day. Caution must be taken however, when ingesting large quantities of fat-soluble vitamins (A, D, E, and K) due to the possibil-ity of toxicity stemming from bodily storage of these vitamins.

MINERALS

Until recently, vitamins were thought to be a more important concern in athletic performance than minerals. Through vast research, it is now believed that minerals play a very significant role in various bodily func-tions and are essential to physical movement. A deficiency in any mineral can be disastrous to peak performance and health. There are basically sev-enty-two minerals that are required for optimum health. Of these seventy-two, the major ones are: calcium, phosphorus, potassium, sodium, chloride, magnesium, and sulfur. Some of the minor minerals are: chromium, cobalt, flouride, zinc, selenium, silicon, boron, iron, copper, iodine, manganese, molybdenum, nickel, arsenic, and vanadium.

Like vitamins, minerals are frequently lacking in most diets. Failure to consume adequate levels of these important substances can result in fatigue, weakness, and injury. Since the stresses associated with sport activ-ities promote the loss of various minerals, it becomes even more important to increase your mineral intake.

WATER

Water is by far the largest single constituent of the body, making up 45 to 80 percent of total body weight. It is the universal medium within which all the body processes work. The major supply of water comes from ingested liquids and foods. A secondary source is called metabolic water and refers to the water that results from the body breaking down chemical bonds.

This amazing substance is involved in every bodily function. A reduc-tion in water means more concentrated blood. Thicker blood is more

Water is healthy living.

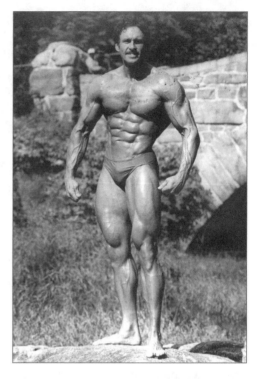

susceptible to clotting, less able to deliver oxygen to your brain and muscles, and less capable of transporting substances to and from your various tissues. Temperature regulation is also controlled by water. This illustrious substance lubricates your joints. It's responsible for the actions involved in energy production, as well as helping the kidneys expel toxins and wastes from the body.

The body has several routes for ridding itself of wastewater. The most frequently used route of fluid output is through the kidneys. Other routes for fluid output include the skin, lungs, and gastrointestinal tract. It is important to maintain adequate fluid levels. Regulating your fluid intake according to thirst is an inefficient method due to the fact that once you're experiencing thirst, you're already dehydrated.

Water is the primary element in all body fluids. Body fluids contain electrolytes. These substances serve three general functions in the body:

- Many are essential minerals (necessary for survival).

- They control the water pressure between body compartments.

- They help maintain the acid/base balance required for normal cellular activity.

Insufficient water intake can result in muscle weakness, headaches, hypertension, and confusion. A 10 percent reduction of water in your body can make you sick; a 20 percent loss of water can mean death.

As an athlete, water helps you recover from your workouts, aids in fat-based fueling of muscles, and provides for storage of water inside your cells. When you become dehydrated, all of these functions are compromised, and your performance levels lower. A reduction in water can result in a drop in physical performance of 20 to 30 percent. As we just cautioned, don't wait until you're thirsty to drink water. By the time your body reaches that point, you are already deficient in this fluid.

The importance of water is unquestionable, especially for anyone who exercises. As the major "ingredient" of the human body, plenty of water is essential to healthy and qualitative athletic performance. Drink between six and eight full glasses of water a day. But don't overdo it. Too much of anything can have adverse effects. This includes water. We urge all our clients not to drink fluoridated water. Why? Because some studies have shown that fluoride may contain higher levels of aluminum, which may increase risk of memory loss and other brain disorders.

YOU NEED A WELL-BALANCED DIET
AND PROPER SUPPLEMENTATION TO EXCEL

Even if you eat a well-balanced diet, you may still have a difficult time replenishing all the vitamins, minerals, and foodstuffs that are used up during exercise and competitions. This is because many of the foods we eat are depleted of important nutrients. Today, farmers deliberately or unknowingly create poor, low-grade soil that is lacking in nutrients through the planting of monocrops, or large fields that are dedicated to a single plant. The soil is further depleted due to the improper balance of organisms brought about by the use of pesticides, weeds, and insecticides. The crops produced in this way have less than adequate nutrition. Whereas forty years ago if you ate one tomato, today, to get the same nutritional value, you would have to eat half a bushel! For maximum effect, certain supplements must be taken at specific times in order to maximize their effects on the body. Usually, this is done during the restorative processes following exercise.

Many people are very conservative in their beliefs and prejudices regarding nutritional practices. Athletes are continually looking for special foods and diets that will help to improve their performance. Unfortunately, many athletes are not knowledgeable about nutrition. Supplementation is often necessary to assure a balanced level of nutrition. Today, the food supplement business has blossomed into an incredible industry, and many great products have been developed.

In addition to using nutritional supplements to replenish the body's energy and resources, supplements should be taken for increased work capacity and a speedier recovery. Stress destroys these vital chemicals. Only through supplementation can we achieve the necessary nutrition for recovery.

A proper combination of food types is critical to supplying ample energy for your particular physical demands and recovery needs. Not all athletes require the same nutrition. But without good nutrition and proper supplementation, you will find it quite difficult to improve on your physical performance.

It is well established that proper eating allows you to excel and be a better competitor. Your diet needs to meet both your energy demand and nutritional requirements. Your diet will be effective only when it meets all the various demands placed on it through physical activity. If you do not meet these demands through your diet, you can easily become extremely fatigued.

As elite athletes know, skill and physical training are just not enough for the competitive edge. An integration of all available training technologies, including proper nutrition, contributes significantly to your peak performance. Without a doubt, athletes have specific dietary needs. Let's see what your needs might be by looking deeper into food and its role in exercise.

Food and Exercise

*A*re you tired of living with pain, weakness, fatigue, or some other nagging condition that either prevents you from enjoying your golf game or even affects the outcome of your game? Are you frustrated that your body just will not perform as you wish? That's why we're so excited to be teaching you about your body, how it works, and how to keep it working. Knowledge is a very effective tool for ending those years of suffering and frustration. You, too, can now experience once and for all the most incredible results from a proper nutritional and exercise program. You no longer have to fall for the myth that you have to be weak and tired unless you do some ridiculously strenuous workout or diet regimen. Basically, all that is required is to learn what the body wants and needs from you. Keep in mind that the body wants to achieve a balance (homeostasis) of all its cells, hormones, systems, and structures.

How do you start? First, you must learn the fundamentals of eating. With

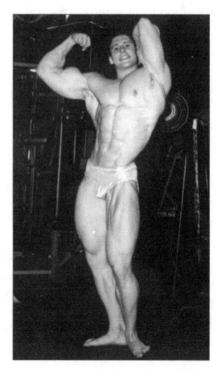

No one has to live with weakness and fatigue.

every bite of food, every intake of fluid, and every breath of air, you're signaling the body to go in and out of homeostasis.

Eating food in a controlled way—that is to say, eating the proper amounts and kinds of foods at the right time, and in the proper combinations—is your ticket to balance. Staying in balance is a matter of knowing the basic rules and principles that the body must follow. The human body does not lead, it follows orders; it does not think, it reacts. Basically, it follows the orders you give it. Some of those orders are given every time you eat or drink. It's that simple. If you follow the rules, you win. By eating the wrong foods, at the wrong time, and in the wrong proportions, you lose.

FALSE DATA ABOUT FOOD

Too often, the way we eat is governed by fad diets or the latest miracle diet, usually promoted by so-called diet experts who promote diet breakthroughs based on false or incorrect information. Not only that, for years the U.S. government's guidelines for eating correctly, summarized in the food pyramid, have been dead wrong. You've been deceived by recommendations promoting a well-balanced diet that includes consuming all the food groups in one meal. These recommendations violate the basic physiology of digestion. In reality, the best and most complete digestion takes place when only one food group at a time is present in the digestive system, as opposed to a variety. (We'll explain the sound physiological reasons for eating foods in compatible combinations later in the chapter.)

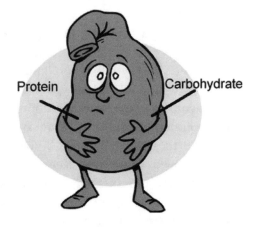

Rather than reason and understanding, confusion and frustration rule. People have gotten to the point where they are desperate, and desperation leads to apathy. But don't despair. There is a message of hope here. Let's continue by taking a closer look at some of these destructive eating habits.

Look at what the majority of us eat. We are "feeding" ourselves with feed. Yes, feed like livestock eats, except in this case we are the livestock.

We feed grains, corn, rice, and potatoes to our cows, pigs, chickens, and other farm animals, and it really fattens them up. Does this diet sound familiar? That's right, it's what the U.S. food pyramid recommends—what the government recommends! Refined flour and grain products (all carbohydrates) make up the majority of our diets. We have become our own farmers. We are the ranchers, and we've been fattening ourselves up. And beware if a label on a product says "fat-free." Read closely. It is sure to be high in carbohydrates. We have all been duped into eating like cows. Look around you. We are a country of people who are shaped and act like livestock—fat and lethargic. Going out and being a great golfer with a pair of hooves is very difficult indeed. As a country, we have spent trillions on health care, billions on research, and yet we're still among the fattest and most out-of-shape cultures on the planet. Something just doesn't add up.

For over two decades now, leading authorities have been telling you that eating a high-protein diet is unnecessary, that eating fat in your diet will kill you, and that a high-carbohydrate diet is ideal. Leading food-industry advertisers have brainwashed you into believing that this low-fat, low-protein, high-carbohydrate diet is the healthiest for you. Tell us then why there is such a high rate of cardiovascular disease, cancer, diabetes, arthritis, and other diet-related diseases? It's time to open your eyes and your mind. We know this is a book about golf, but let's face it—it's hard to play golf if you're dead.

People with fat, out-of-shape bodies, and unbalanced body chemistries have become epidemic in our society. Let's examine the relationship of what you eat and how it affects you. The following are some basic diet myths you should know:

- **Myth 1:** Eating food with fewer calories will help you lose weight. Wrong. Starving yourself will only slow down your metabolism. It will lead to muscle and bone loss, and you will simply increase your levels of fat and fatigue. Every time you make a reduction in your daily calorie intake, your body resets its metabolism to compensate. Not a good scenario on the golf course.

- **Myth 2:** All fats are bad for you. Wrong. There are bad fats that should be avoided in your diet, and there are good fats that should be consumed. The good fats can actually help clean out bad body fats. Conjugated linoleic acid (CLA) and the omega-3, -6, and -9 fats are examples of good fats.
  Here's why. CLA is found in small amounts mainly in meat and dairy

products. CLA has been shown to increase muscle mass while reducing body fat. Studies have also shown it has remarkable anticatabolic, antioxidant, and immune-enhancing benefits. CLA may be the most significant nutrient discovered in this decade. With anticatabolic effects rivaling even the strongest pharmaceutical compounds, CLA is a naturally occurring nutrient with the ability to help you pack on lean muscle and reduce body fat. It also possesses health-promoting properties.

The omega-3, -6, and -9 fatty acids regulate oxygen use, electron transport, and energy production. These fats are abundant in certain foods such as fish, nuts, and avocados. They can enhance lipolysis (body-fat breakdown) and decrease lipogenesis (body-fat formation). The combined breakdown of stored body fat and decrease in additional body fat formation can have very positive results for the dieter. You actually end up making less and breaking down more body fat when using these oils.

Also, for your information, low-fat diets trigger a scarcity of fat in the body, which leads to excess fat storage. The body will also convert other foods to fat in a desperate attempt to supplement the missing fat.

- **Myth 3:** Crackpot diets may work. Wrong. Crackpot diets like the cabbage diet where you eat nothing but cabbage, or the water diet where you drink water a billion times a day, simply do not work. They are just silly attempts to cover up the truth. Diuretics, colonics, or diets based on shakes, bars, pills, creams, the so-called Hollywood actors' diet, the Subway diet, you name it—they will just lead you down the path to disaster.

Conventional doctors, nutritionists, and dietitians will often steer you down the pathway to destruction. Though they are well intentioned, they are usually ill informed. If you want to increase the efficiency of your golf game and have a stronger, healthier body and mind, stay out of this maze of misinformation.

YOU ARE WHAT YOU CONSUME

Every type of athlete needs to be in shape. They need to have an endless supply of energy to feel good. A lean, muscular body, produced by eating correctly will help you achieve these goals. Staying out of a slump in your golf game means also keeping your body's key hormone levels in balance. You can balance your hormone levels with proper diet and exercise. Your hormones, along with the nervous system, are the command centers of the body. They regulate almost all functions.

The nutrients in protein, carbohydrates, and fats generate a hormonal response that can affect how you feel, think, and act. Knowing how to control these macronutrients is the gateway to real power. Every time you step out on a golf course or a driving range, millions of tiny cells go into action or inaction, depending on your cellular condition. This cellular condition depends greatly on your ability to feed and supplement those cells.

Food is a controlling force in the body. Eating foods correctly in the right combinations, and understanding the principles of digestion and how those principles affect your emotions (via the hormones), will go a long way in helping you perfect and maintain your body.

Let's make a simple analogy to a computer. Food is the software, and the body is the hardware. Putting in a certain type of food will activate a specific software program. The food will stimulate certain cellular activity, and that will affect how that food plays out in your body. Every food activates a different program, and different combinations of foods will cause different effects also. What you put in your mouth by your own hand will determine your fate.

The absorption, digestion, and utilization of these macronutrients are governed by the laws of science and chemistry. These laws determine what happens in between the food going in and the food coming out. Just take a little time to learn the basics about food digestion. It will help you understand how eating the wrong foods could sabotage your game!

THE BASICS OF DIGESTION

Digestion is the act of breaking down food to obtain its component parts, including energy, water, and nutrients. The energies in food are needed by every cell and organ in the body. These energies are vital to your well-being and to your performance in life and on the golf course. You are what you consume. If you don't consume correctly, you will be consumed. Many die of hunger, but many more die from eating.

The digestive tract varies its digestive fluids and enzymes in the presence of different types of food. In order for the foods to be digested and absorbed easier, these variations must include changes in fluid pH levels and enzymes. Some foods require a more acidic environment, other foods a more alkaline environment. Different foods also require different amounts of different enzymes. Protein digestion, for example, begins in the stomach and requires an acid base and acid secretions such as hydrochloric acid and the enzyme pepsin. Carbohydrate and starch digestion begins in the mouth and requires an alkaline base and alkaline digestive secretions—and none of these work well together.

If you mix these two (acid/alkaline) together, they neutralize each other and offset the efficiency and potency of each other. Have you ever seen the old magic trick where the magician pours blue fluids (acids) into a cup of red fluid (alkaline) and the solution turns clear? When you mix an acid with an alkaline, it turns to water. Food *cannot* be digested in water. Therefore, attempting to play golf with a stomach full of partially digested acidic and alkaline foods is certainly a less than optimum condition. Food left in water will rot. Now imagine that inside you—it's bound to affect your golf game. This condition causes bloating, gas, and indigestion, and will rob you of energy and throw off your concentration and timing.

Matching the correct fluids and enzymes to the type of food eaten is critical. These factors can only work properly when the character of the foods is similar. Dissimilar foods such as bread and cheese disrupt digestive efficiency. Natural food combinations that contain both protein and carbohydrates, as in some whole grains, are digested more easily and efficiently because nature has provided most (but not all) enzymes in the food to aid the digestive system. It is the more common combinations such as meat and flour (as in the typical sandwich) that cause most of the problems.

In a sense, we subject ourselves to digestive poisoning when we mix the wrong kinds of foods. Most people do not eat one food type at a time (per meal). For example, most people don't eat meat and follow it with a carbohydrate or starch. Instead, they tend to eat these foods together in meals that include meats and potatoes, toast and eggs, and so on. As far back as biblical times, eating protein separately from carbohydrates was the law. Even then, people knew that the process of digesting two separate types of food was not optimum. The digestive system was just not built efficiently enough to handle the processing and absorption of protein and carbohydrates together. Now take time to think about this, as it is contrary to what you have been led to believe and we're sure contrary to what you're currently doing. Tests have shown a large amount of undigested starch in the stools of people who mix their protein and carbohydrates together. Undigested food wastes energy and nutrients.

Today, people take indigestion for granted. Bloating, gas, stomach pains, and so on are considered normal. They're not! They're real danger signals. And how does society handle these danger signals? We do it with over-the-counter medications like Alka-Seltzer, Tums, or Pepto-Bismol. Wake up! You're killing yourself. You're living deep under the cloak of the food phantom, where knowledge lives in shadows.

The human body can endure most anything, and will try in desperation to adapt to even the worst conditions. It is this adaptation that uses up so much energy and can leave you tired and confused and certainly less efficient at any game. It is not only an inefficient way of eating, but also it shortchanges the body of the nutrition it critically needs. It stands to reason then that the best meals are the simplest ones where proteins, carbohydrates, and fats are ingested separately.

BASICS GUIDELINES FOR PROPER FOOD COMBINING

Basically, food combining is a question of timing. The less complex the food, the less time it takes to break down in the digestive tract. Fruits and simple sugars are digested quickly, vegetables relatively quickly. Grains take more time, and oils and heavy proteins take the most time. It's best to avoid combining foods that are digested quickly with those that take a long time to digest.

Following are the basic rules of proper food combining:

1. Eat acids (fruits) and starches (pasta, rice) separately. Acids neutralize the alkaline environment required for the digestion of starch and result in fermentation and indigestion.

2. Eat proteins and carbohydrates at separate meals. Proteins require an acidic environment for digestion.

3. Do not eat more than one type of protein per meal.

4. Eat proteins and acidic foods at separate meals. Acidic foods inhibit the secretion of the digestive acids required for protein digestion. Undigested protein putrefies and produces some potent poisons.

5. Eat fats and proteins at separate meals. Fats slow down the digestive process. Some foods, especially nuts with over 50 percent fat, require hours for complete digestion.

6. Eat sugars (fruits) and proteins at separate meals.

7. Eats sugars (fruits) and starchy foods at separate meals. Fruits require no digestion in the stomach and are held up if they are eaten with foods requiring digestion.

8. Eat melons alone. They combine with almost no other food.

9. Skip the desserts. They lie heavy in the stomach, require no digestion, and simply ferment.

Avoid drinking fluids with meals. Drinking while eating will dilute your saliva and lessen the efficiency of starch digestion. Also, it can weaken the digestive fluids and enzymes found in the stomach. Drinking fluids is best done between meals. Aim not to drink one-half hour before a meal or one and a half hours after. Try to limit fluid intake to sipping if you find you must have fluids while eating.

The lists of foods on page 95 will help get you started planning meals with proper food combinations. The diagram further explains which food groups may or may not be combined. The gray arrows show proper food combining, and the black arrows indicate which food groups should be separated.

Volumes have been written about which foods should be eaten together and which combinations should be avoided to maximize nutrition and minimize indigestion. Check out your local bookstore or library for more information on food combining.

ESTABLISH AN EATING SCHEDULE

All of nature works in cycles or rhythms, and so too does the human body—except, that is, when humans intervene and follow the pattern of hunger and gluttony. The rhythms of the body tie into every function we do. The process of digesting is a good example. The digestive rhythms have a limited supply of digestive enzymes flowing. These enzymes have their maximum effect, and are present in greater amounts, while you are eating. Once you finish eating, the supply of digestive enzymes dwindles. For this reason, time must be allowed between meals for the digestive system to kick in again. This takes us to our next issue—regularity. In other words, when is the best time to eat foods from each food group, how much, and how often?

Most people eat whenever they find time within the framework of a

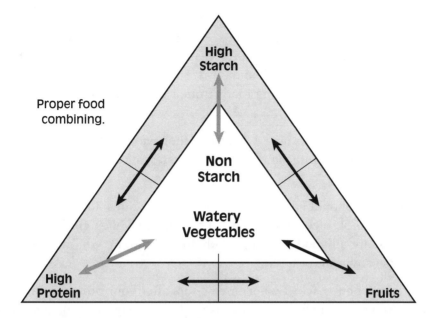

Foods High in Starch

Avocados
Carrots
Corn
Eggplant
Grains
Pastas
Potatoes (all)
Rice
Squash
Turnips

Non-Starchy Vegetables (High Water Content)

Artichokes
Asparagus
Broccoli
Brussels sprouts
Cabbage
Cauliflower
Celery
Cucumbers
Endive
Green beans
Green leafy
  vegetables
Okra
Parsley
Peppers (all)
Sea vegetables
Swiss chard
Zucchini

Foods High in Protein

Beans
Dairy products
Fish
Legumes
Poultry
Meat (all)
Nuts
Seafood
Seeds
Wild game

Fruits

Apples
Apricots
Bananas
Berries
Cherries
Figs
Grapefruits
Lemons
Melons (all)
Nectarines
Oranges
Peaches
Pears
Pineapples
Plums
Tomatoes

three-meal day. But basically it's ideal to eat with regularity, at the same time each day, and in small amounts, altering the type of food eaten each meal. There are also physiological reasons for eating particular food groups at different times of the day, as the body's energy requirements vary. The best times for eating foods from a particular food group are as follows:

- **Morning:** In the morning when you first wake up, the body needs energy. At this point, complex carbohydrates, such as oatmeal, should eaten.

- **Lunch:** You should have a protein meal two or three hours later, and it should consist solely of one kind of protein. Egg whites, chicken, turkey, and fish are all good choices. If you are vegetarian, you may want to consider soybeans or tofu.

- **Midafternoon snack:** Two or three hours after your protein meal, you should have a small snack, such as fruit. Fruit requires little digestion and should be eaten alone.

- **Dinner:** The last meal of the day should be a light protein meal of some sort. During the night, specifically one and a half hours into sleep, the human body rebuilds all tissue. Then, about one and a half hours before awakening, the body shuts down this mechanism and goes into energy production.

You can learn to consume protein, carbohydrates, and fats to your advantage before a competition or golf outing as well. Here are some tips for optimum ways to use these macronutrients before events.

Protein Use

Generally, protein should not be eaten before a competition or golf outing because it is a dense molecule and hard to digest. Blood is required for digestion, and the blood, which would ordinarily go toward the performance, will now be trapped in the digestive system and redirected away from the muscle. Remember, it is the muscles that swing the club, and it is the blood that provides the oxygen and energy needed by the body. Equally important are the oxygen and nutrients needed by the brain.

Tests have shown that the optimum time to consume protein is about an hour after your game or exercise session, and anywhere between one to two hours before bedtime. Protein works best for healing and building with human growth hormone, which is excreted midway through your sleep. The timing is mutually perfect for both, as it takes approximately four hours to digest protein, as well as to release human growth hormone.

It is best to eat carbohydrates two hours prior to your game or exercise session, and also right after. This is because the carbohydrates will have a protein-sparing effect on the muscle. They will be burned first as fuel instead of the protein, thus sparing the protein for building, healing, and raising the body's metabolism.

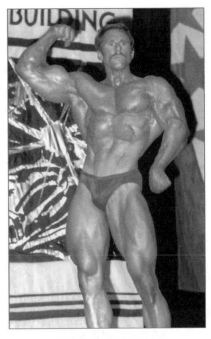

Protein is muscle, muscle is power.

Your protein need increases as stress increases. Mental stress, especially, increases the need for protein. Our daily recommendation is one gram of protein per pound of body weight, and approximately 1.42 grams during stressful times, such as prior to a golf match or tournament.

Carbohydrate Use

Carbohydrates are the primary source of energy. How fast the body's supply of energy is depleted depends on the type of carbohydrate consumed. Refined carbohydrates release and deplete quickly, while more complex carbohydrates convert to glucose and are used up more slowly. Carbohydrates are best eaten after intense activity when the body needs energy.

If you find it difficult to maintain your energy level on the golf course, you may be suffering from sugar withdrawal, where your supply of stored sugar simply runs out, followed shortly after by disorientation and fatigue. You can kiss that par or birdie good-bye. Helping your body store as much glycogen (stored glucose) as possible, for as many rounds of golf as possible, can only enhance your performance, calm the body, and free the mind.

The best way to achieve this is by combining the correct carbohydrate intake with high-intensity exercise. (We will get into high-intensity exercise in the following chapter.) In short, the theory is as follows: three days prior to your golf outing, exercise hard enough to deplete the glycogen in the muscle. Any exercise that uses high-volume resistance will inevitably deplete glycogen sources in the muscle. Then, after training, rest the body while eating a considerable amount of complex carbohydrates. Eat between forty and eighty grams of complex carbohydrates every two to three hours. Be sure to drink sufficient amounts of water (at least eight to ten glasses), as the water helps to store the carbohydrates. We recommend you try this before you go golfing to find out exactly how the carbohydrates affect you.

Fat Use

Fats are a good secondary source of energy. Though we do not recommend eating many fats, good sources of unsaturated fat can be eaten with a protein source from time to time. Good fats are conducive to the absorption of protein, but bad fats are not. Remember not to combine fats with starches and fruits.

ONE LAST CAVEAT

Eating too much is equally as destructive as eating the wrong combination of foods. Consuming more than your body needs can lead to obesity, indigestion, and gastric diseases. Food advertisers have convinced us that our eyes are big enough for our mouths because, unfortunately, everything we see, we usually eat. The solution to this dilemma is simple: eat smaller portions more often.

Now that you know what nutrients the body wants and needs, let's see how exercise can help you fine tune this machine.

10

Cardiovascular Fitness and Weight Training

*B*eware of gimmicks. There are more exercise devices and quack inventions in the fitness field for golf than ever. The very people who claim to be advancing the fields of exercise, sports training, and fitness have all but destroyed them. Just because some celebrity endorses a product or demonstrates it in an infomercial does not validate the product. These devices or routines are an insult to your intelligence. Likewise, just because some world-class athlete endorses an exercise product doesn't lend it credibility. So, if a great pro golfer is suddenly using some club, ball, or other golfing device, and they claim it has helped them win a tournament or two, can you believe it? We don't think so. Most developed their skill long before any of these devices were invented! Having become recognized as a golf star, many athletes become "instant experts" on practically everything.

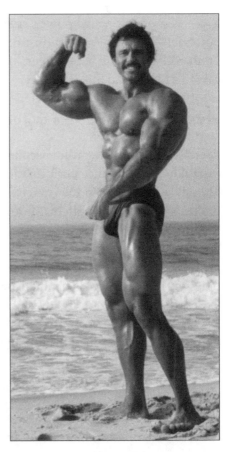

Muscle machine.

It is a mistake to listen to such people who seldom, if ever, really understand the actual cause-and-effect relationship responsible for effective physical conditioning. Doubly unfortunate is that almost none of the published information is based on scientifically demonstrated data. If God made idiots as a working model, then fitness experts are the finished product.

Exercise is a science. It is the study of how the body responds to a particular goal or task. The goal of our exercise program is to build a better body—a better machine—that will work in an explosive way with agility, flexibility, balance, stamina, and strength. Our program can also bring harmony to the body and will quiet the noise in your head so you can handle stress (both known and unknown). It will help prevent injury and ward off disease, lower body fat, raise muscle tone, and it will allow you to tap into a reservoir of untouched power, enabling you to use your body to its fullest potential—beyond your wildest dreams. In a nutshell, our exercise program will allow you access to an arsenal of physiological and psychological tools that, up to this point, have been lost to you.

FITNESS IN GOLF *IS* AN ASSET

Exercise, specifically cardiovascular exercise and weight training, are successful tools to enhance performance in all sports, and golf is no exception. Though a latecomer to the exercise community, golf fitness is becoming a top priority for many golfers. More and more top golfers are using exercise to improve their games. (In a moment, we will look into what some of the top players are doing to tap into their potential.) Exercise, when done correctly with the proper routine, can bring about incredible results. In our opinion, the problem is that no one in authority is quite sure how to approach exercise for golf.

We have traveled countless miles throughout the United States observing exercise facilities in both clubs and tournaments with much disappointment. We have also studied many books and manuals on the subject of exercise for golfers, and we can come to only one conclusion: golfers need help. Their exercise trainers need help, and the entire field of exercise for golfers, in our opinion, is a joke. Not only is the lack of exercise an area of concern for golfers, but so is the proper exercise that will not hinder the golfer.

Historical records indicate that the advent of the game required that after a friendly round of golf, all the participants would ceremonially gather and share in a barrel (keg) of beer. Times haven't changed much as alcohol is a common sight after a day on the links, with the winners celebrating and the losers drowning their sorrows. It seems that this tradition of destroying the body has trapped many over the years.

Smoking, alcohol, prescription drugs, and steroids, as well as hard-core drug use such as marijuana, cocaine, and heroine, have infiltrated major tours for both men and women over the years. There is even a trend that started in the late 1980s of sport psychologists prescribing prescription drugs like beta-blockers, Valium, and Ritalin to top players around the world. It's all a futile attempt to improve their game, when the truth of the matter is all of these products taken in enough quantity will *kill you!*

It was well known that players such as the American golfer Ben Hogan would light up cigarettes on the course. In fact, Mr. Hogan did promotional work for a cigarette manufacturer. Nowadays, tournament professionals and the local club pros have turned into twelve-step alcoholics and tell stories of what they could have been.

THE FITNESS BUZZ

An attempt to bring the body's role and function into the mainstream was initiated by Frank Stranahan, one of the world's most prolific amateur golf champions, and Gary Player, a South African professional golfer, in the 1950s and 1960s. These two made the first real efforts at conditioning the body to enhance their play. Other professionals and the general public heckled their efforts, claiming that they would ruin their swing because golfers didn't need muscles to hit a ball and conditioning was not important. After all, all they were doing was walking.

Since that time, very little changed until a fit guy by the name of Eldrick "Tiger" Woods came around and started cleaning everybody's clock. All of a sudden, people started deciding that fitness could be an asset after all and wanted to get into shape. But this posed a new dilemma. How so?

With the financial growth of the Professional Golfers' Association (PGA) Tour in the 1980s and 1990s, players have been well catered to off the course. Club manufacturers provide trailers to give away free clubs; swing gurus with camcorders are ready and waiting to provide free advice; and seldom-used fitness trailers can be found next to the driving range, complete with their own personal trainers. Yet today's players remain fat, weak, and out of shape.

A few years back, we ventured into one of these fitness trailers to find one player reading while on a bicycle. Another was doing some forearm curls with "massive" three-pound weights, while yet another player was stretched out by the physical therapist. There was no fat being burned! No muscle being built here! In fact, there wasn't a bead of sweat being dripped by anyone other than us, and we had just come into the air-conditioned environment from the ninety-degree heat! So it was no surprise to us that when we entered the trailer, obviously fit and strong, the trainer started getting nervous because we were in the condition the players wanted to be but weren't achieving with their weekend-certified personal trainers.

An article in *Golf Magazine* (2001) that was written around the same time discussed a few fitness trendsetters of the PGA Tour, describing their workout routines.

The Swedish professional golfer Jesper Parnevik has been well known for his eccentricity ever since he touted eating lava ash to cleanse his body and then switched over to an all-fruit diet. His effort at getting into shape involved a split-day workout routine with a morning of running, medicine ball work, and light weights, followed by a slightly more intense workout in the evening and some additional running.

Australian Stuart Appleby, who ranks as one of the longer hitters on the tour, has strived to be quicker, faster, and more flexible over the years. His regimen includes riding a stationary bike for forty-five minutes to burn fat and boost leg strength. His general weight routine includes bench presses, squats, arms, shoulders and stomach work (limiting everything to above the hips), as well as lifting weights to stabilize the small muscles and simulating golf motions.

Years ago, American golfer Rocco Mediate was fat and overweight at a whopping 250 pounds. It got so bad that in 1993, because of his condition, surgery was required to repair a fractured disc in his lower back. Determined to recover, Rocco began a fitness regimen that included aerobics, light weight-lifting with many repetitions, and plenty of abdominal work. It took five long years to achieve his current weight of 185 pounds. Currently, Rocco has said he has replaced the weight training with Pilates-type exercises.

Unlike others who have jumped on the new bandwagon of fitness, Grant Waite from New Zealand has long been employing good nutrition coupled with all types of fitness regimens, including plyometrics (a type of explosive exercise that uses movements to develop muscular power), stretching, weights, and even yoga, to improve his conditioning.

Though some of the top ten players, such as American Phil Mickelson and South African Ernie Els, have openly said how they despise physical fitness, it is clearly evident that the fitness buzz has picked up with a substantial number of players preaching the benefits.

We truly applaud all of those who have recognized the benefits of fitness. We only wish that their efforts were used more productively, as effort alone does not always breed success or champions. In this chapter, you will learn how exercising improperly or without intensity will do little to nothing to change your current condition. It is time to find out exactly why fitness should be incorporated into the lifestyle of all golfers, what the popular myths about exercise and golf are, and how to get the correct results.

WHAT THE ATOMIC GOLF SYSTEM WILL DO FOR YOU

Why is the Atomic Golf System necessary? Because it is impossible to realize your full potential on the golf course without a planned program of exercise, strength, stamina, flexibility, and mental toughness. Golfers are often called upon to endure stresses not ordinarily connected with life. They are required to deliver force, speed, and accuracy, time after time on the golf course, sometimes for days on end. This requires physical fitness, which means that the player needs to be at the highest levels of conditioning. Anything below this standard can only encourage poor health, aches and pains, premature aging, and lots of bogeys. Therefore, a properly planned program of exercise is essential for optimal play, regardless of your age or sex.

An exercise routine that promotes cardiovascular and muscular endurance with aerobic and anaerobic conditioning provides the fastest and most effective way to improve your physical and mental health. You can expect:

- Higher energy levels
- Improved digestion
- Weight control
- Bone and muscle growth
- Emotional relief

• Heart protection

And unless your body is in optimal condition, you will have little success in achieving your goals in your game. Let's get started.

WHY CARDIO-CONDITIONING IS A MUST

Aerobic fitness refers to exercise that puts oxygen demands upon the body. These demands, over a prolonged period of time, will bring about a change in the body's ability to handle oxygen. These changes occur mainly in the lungs, heart, and vascular system. The term *aerobic* means the utilization of oxygen. Oxygen is a catalyst for burning fat—a key component of getting in shape.

Aerobic fitness involves endurance-type activities. The key to aerobic fitness is not intensity, but duration—constant, steady activity over a sustained period of time. It's not hard work that counts in aerobic exercise, but the building up of endurance over time and distance. When people attempt to make their aerobic activity more challenging by running or walking up hills, or carrying hand or ankle weights, they are defeating the purpose, for the harder the exercise, the more anaerobic it becomes. Anaerobic exercise builds muscle and bone, but does little for the heart and lungs. It shuts down the fat-burning process for a more efficient source of energy—sugar.

You can burn a greater amount of fat playing with a yo-yo than climbing a mountain. This may sound preposterous, but it's true. The reason for this is because all calories are not the same. It's a fact that the harder you work at burning fat, the less fat you burn. To understand this concept you need to understand fat and how it is burned.

Fat Burning

Fat is actually an incredible substance that is made by the body and stored in times of plenty. Fat has a mind of its own. It loves itself, but it's often very lonely and wants plenty of friends. It doesn't care who you are or what you do. Fat prefers those who do little and eat a lot. You think fat's bad; fat thinks it's good. "Pile it on" is fat's motto. The more the merrier. As a matter of fact, fat loves you. It's concerned for your welfare. Fat actually believes you're going to starve someday, so it tries to protect you. Fat does this by accumulating in deposit areas around the body. Generally, it tends to accumulate in the areas of little use. Fat is a tenant that doesn't like noisy, high-traffic housing—it prefers the quiet life.

Fat deposits are made from calories that are eaten in excess of your energy output. It is a simple matter of supply and demand. If you balance input versus output, fat will not accumulate. When you eat more than your body needs or can process into tissue, the excess is converted into fat. Simply put, fat is stored energy. If you don't burn it, you store it. Energy is the most valuable element in your body. Energy keeps your heart, lungs, and cells going. It drives the brain, liver, and so on. Energy is so valuable, in fact, that if the body has a chance to store it, it will. However, all bodies are not created equal. Some bodies store fat more easily than others. Some bodies have more fat cells and fat deposit sites than others. It sounds unfair, and it is.

Scientists believe that the first few years of your life are when you accumulate not only fat deposit sites, but also the number of fat cells in those sites. Others believe genetics are responsible. We feel it's a combination of both: bad luck and bad habits.

The body is always burning fat at some rate, but if your goal is to decrease body fat, you have to increase your fat-burning activity. Generally, during aerobic exercise, the body burns carbohydrates for the first twenty minutes. After it has exhausted this reserve of energy, it will go to its alternative source—fat. This is why we believe the first twenty minutes of aerobic exercise is an absolute waste of time. In order to begin burning fat immediately in your cardio-routine, you should do some anaerobic activity first. Exercises such as curls or squats will exhaust your sugar reserves, thereby allowing you to immediately begin burning fat with your aerobic training. If you burn off the carbs first, then your body will be ready to burn fat. Once you're in this fat-burning mode, your metabolism will stay elevated, even when the exercise is over.

Why is it so important to keep your metabolism elevated? Remember, metabolism is a set of complicated cellular actions that are always running. It's the inner machinery that distributes and regulates body mechanics such as hormone secretion, fat burning, respiration, recovery from illness, and so on. Exercise increases the efficiency of the metabolism. It's a fact that individuals with a high ratio of muscle to fat basically have a better metabolism. This allows for better and more efficient distribution of food.

Muscles are like mini-furnaces that burn fat. The more toned a muscle, the more efficient it is at burning fuel, in this case, fat. The argument that you should lose weight before beginning a workout program is preposterous. The goal should never be to simply lose weight. You have some good stuff in there, including bones, muscles, organs, tissue, and water. What you want to lose is excess fat, not the good stuff. If you simply attempt aerobics or dieting without toning your body, you will lose muscle. Approximately 20 percent of muscle is lost when you diet or do aerobics alone without anaerobic activity. That equals a 20 percent loss in your ability to burn fat. Therefore, losing weight without toning muscle creates a substantial decrease in your body's fat-burning capacity, and that's nuts! This is the primary cause of the so-called yo-yo effect of most diet plans. Yes, you lose weight, and some of that is fat, but a lot of that is good-quality muscle tissue and water.

Although genetics do play a part in the body's ability to lose or store fat, research shows that anyone can increase their metabolism with exercise. Age has little influence on metabolism, except where the muscles have atrophied. Whether you're a senior or an out-of-shape youngster, it's the percentage of lean muscle that drives the metabolism. It's a simple formula: less activity equals less muscle, equaling a slower metabolism, which means increased fat storage and body decay.

Cardio Conditioning and Fat Burning

There's a lot of confusion regarding the relationship between cardio exercise and fat burning. Let us clear this up for you quickly. If the activity you are performing causes your muscles to exert themselves, more than likely your body is burning sugars or carbohydrates instead of fat. If the activity is of a low order of intensity, for a prolonged period of time, you will more than likely burn fat. Basically, here's why.

The sugar molecule is small and readily available to be transported to a muscle. For example, if you needed to get out of the way of a speeding car, the muscles would have to respond quickly. Instant access to energy would be required. No matter whether physical or emotional, the key is stress. The harder you work, or the more intense the activity, the more sugar you burn.

Fat, as we've said, is a secondary source of energy for the body. It is a much larger and lazier molecule. It has to be gently coaxed into use. Fat does not respond to stress. This is why you can burn more fat playing with a yo-yo than by climbing a mountain. Intensity builds muscle; longevity burns fat.

Keys to successful fat burning include the following:

- Change venues every fat-burning session. For example, use different equipment, such as a treadmill, bike, and so forth, if available. Aim to use all the different venues available to you.

- Vary your time and speed at each session. The human body adapts quickly to any kind of activity it does on a regular basis. Some kind of change in fat-burning activity is necessary to fool the body and stay ahead of its ability to adapt.

How do I know if I'm burning fat, you ask? The following are some helpful hints to answer this question:

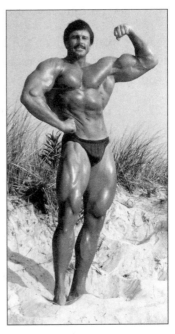

- If your muscles fatigue during aerobic sessions, you're not burning fat.

- If your muscles are sore after aerobic sessions, you're not burning fat. Muscle fatigue and soreness are indicators that your body is using sugar for energy rather than fat. Soreness indicates the presence of lactic acid, which is partially burned sugar, not fat.

To be effective, fat burning should seem ridiculously easy. And one more thing, those aerobic classes where everyone is moving in unison to the sound of music, repetitively, like robots, are absolutely and totally useless for burning fat! They burn calories but not fat.

A strong heart and a lean body are the result of intelligent exercise.

Cardio-Conditioning—Do It Daily!

Contrary to what people think, doing some sort of aerobic activity should be a daily commitment. Aim to exercise for no less than twenty minutes but no more than sixty minutes a day. However, if you are also training with weights (discussed next), you can get all the fitness and conditioning benefits from thirty to forty minutes, three times a week. You can choose whatever aerobic activity you like. Walking or jogging outdoors is best, but a stationary bike or treadmill will do just fine. Start out slow and gradually build up your time and pace. Swimming is also excellent as long as you follow the fat-burning rules—low-intensity exercise over a sustained period of time.

To get the maximum benefit from your aerobic workouts, it is necessary to maintain a sufficient heart rate that relates to you. To figure this out, the following heart-rate formula has been developed:

220 – your age =
100 percent of your ideal rate.

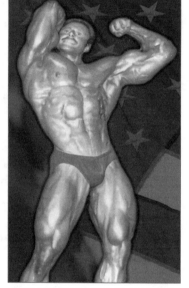

For example, let's apply this formula to a forty-year-old person. The equation would be:

220 – 40 (the age of the individual) = 180

In this case, 180 would be 100 percent of the person's preferred heart rate. However, a less intense percentage of 60 percent may be desired, depending on a person's level of fitness. In this case, the same formula would apply, but the result (220 – 40 = 180) would be multiplied by the desired percentage following. For example:

Not everyone has to look like Mr. Universe.

$$180 \times 0.60 \text{ percent} = 108$$

This individual's targeted heart rate would then be 180 beats per minute. A heart monitor is recommended for a more accurate reading.

In addition to building endurance and burning fat with aerobic exercise, a well-balanced exercise program also requires resistance training for developing your power.

WHY WEIGHT TRAINING IS A MUST

From my (Michael) personal experience, I was once an out-of-shape golfer with no muscle. I went through the same fears and apprehensions that all golfers face when confronted with building muscle. But I was pleasantly surprised and elated that not only was I more fit and leaner, but also I put on sixty pounds of natural muscle and had more power, confidence, and ability than I could possibly have had before. I am forever grateful that I had the knowledge, foresight, and wisdom to let Mr. America (Steve) convince me that it would work.

How does weight training build your muscles? To fully understand how resistance training works, it is necessary to understand the physical structure of muscle tissue and how this structure is altered by weight training.

The Properties and Function of Muscle

The primary function of muscle is to move levers called bones, which then create motion. There are more than six hundred muscles in the human body, accounting for between 40 to 50 percent of body weight. Muscle can strengthen and align your structure, assuring you proper posture. Good posture is one of the most important roles of muscle. It is, after all, your frame and structure on which all else depends. A good, sound structure provides the body with the necessary balance it needs to perform tasks easily. Your entire body works under the principles of balance. Poor muscle tone is the main ingredient of a collapsing structure, leading to poor posture, a loss of balance, and an aberrative swing. Moreover, a weak structure can lead to arthritis and other conditions, and it can shorten a golf career. It is important for anyone who wishes to add as many years as possible to their game—and life—not to overlook an exercise program that will ensure structural balance.

Muscles are made up fibers. These fiber tissues are strands woven together to create a whole mass. What may appear to be a single bulging muscle is, in fact, a great number of tissue fibers. In terms of size, the thicker muscles of the body, such as the thighs and back, have much larger quantities of these fibers than the smaller muscles of the arms and shoulders—and not only are these fibers thicker and heavier, they are also far more numerous.

There are three types of fiber: fast for strength; slow for endurance; and intermediate for a combination of both. Each of us is born with a different ratio of each type, and that is what makes us different. These three types of muscle fiber work side by side and perform different functions. The percentage of the type of fiber you have varies from person to person and from muscle group to muscle group. Neurologists have stated that the activity level of a baby before birth, and then again after interacting with

The Properties of Muscle

- Muscle accomplishes movement by its ability to lengthen and shorten, to recruit fiber to complete a task—the greater the demand, the greater the recruitment.

- This recruitment produces movement by exerting force on tendons that then pull on bones.

- All muscles pull via a joint.

- Strength is the coordinated effort of muscles pulling and working together.

- Muscle pulls from its origin, where it starts, to its insertion, where it finishes.

- All muscles have opposing muscles; movers and opposers work together to create control.

- Balance (synergy) between the mover and the opposer creates the greatest effect of movement.

- Muscle tone equals the degree of constant muscle readiness, which equals explosive power, enduring stamina, and strength.

- This leads to speed over a range of motion (i.e., your golf swing), which equals force.

- Force equals torque.

- Torque equals power.

- Power monitors control.

- Control monitors ability.

- Ability is the precursor to skill.

- Skill in exercise produces the optimum effect.

Please read this as many times as necessary to fully understand the nature and motion of muscle.

the environment, stimulates the brain to produce a certain type of muscle fiber. After the body matures, it is believed you are stuck with that percentage of fiber. But we believe muscle fiber can be altered, or customized, if you will, to act like a more "preferred fiber" better suited for the activity you are engaged in—in this case, golf. Some muscle fibers are better suited than others for increasing your mechanical advantage (the factor by which a mechanism multiplies the force put into it). Mechanical advantage in golf is of utmost importance when hitting a ball.

When you use weights to build up and strengthen your muscles, good things occur. The term "pumped up" refers to the swelling surrounding the muscle being worked, which is due to rapidly increasing blood flow into that area. The body always sends a fresh supply of blood to any area of exertion to supply the working area with the nutrients and oxygen needed to carry out its function, while also carrying away broken-down cells from that area so the nutrients can build up and help the area become stronger and more useful.

Your body has been designed to meet the demands placed on it. When any level of resistance is placed on a muscle, the body sets up an existing level of muscle development. The existing level of development can be changed by using the Atomic Golf System of training, which causes muscles to overload and tear down in response to the demand placed on them. As this happens, the body will receive a signal to rush nutrients and oxygen to this particular area of stress. The muscle then swells with nutrients. Since your body knows its business, it sends more than is needed to rebuild this broken-down tissue.

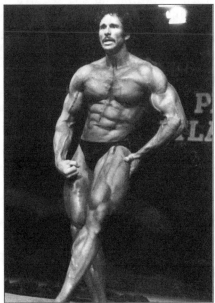

There is *no* substitute for hard work.

This condition should occur after several repetitions of any given exercise, and it is what is referred to as pumped up. A note to remember is that the breaking down of tissue will occur only when you "overwork" your existing level of development. If you don't, then you're only doing what your body is already capable of, and no message will be sent to relieve it with nutrients and rebuilding materials.

You must have maximum intensity to stimulate maximum growth. Maximum intensity does not refer to using excessive amounts of weight, but rather to exerting the greatest effort with force and speed in the short-est amount of time. It is not necessary to train in a dangerous fashion, using heavy weights, to attain maximum-possible intensity.

A well-toned muscle will have a tremendous amount of preload capacity (potential energy), thus increasing your mechanical advantage. You can gain a mechanical advantage by performing one of the following five actions:

- Muscles that are the *prime movers* (the ones most involved in the swing) produce the most force.

- *Assistant movers* help the prime movers (the ones most involved in the swing).

- The opposing muscles set up torque, which is the measure of how much of that opposing force is acted upon the object. This creates power. These opposing muscles are called *antagonists.*

- *Stabilizer muscles* stabilize skeletal structure and bone to keep you steady and focused.

- *True and helping* synergists (muscles that coordinate both the prime movers and the antagonists) are watchdogs over prime movers.

To familiarize yourself with the array of ways the body can move, see the inset "A Primer on Movement" on page 113.

False Data and Specialized Golf Workouts

Not all exercise programs are good or correct. Quite frankly, there are few exercise programs on the market that are designed for golf. Most of these exercise programs are designed to target the so-called golf muscles, but not every muscle. An exercise routine must be designed to work areas from your toes to your head, and it must work in a synergy of motion. By focus-ing only on specific areas, you make things worse by creating imbalance. This is the last thing you want to do.

An incorrect exercise routine will disrupt your natural swing. These routines cause imbalances to occur in the muscular system, causing some muscles to get strong while allowing others to atrophy. Only when you have built and maintained all of the major muscular groups will the deli-cate balance of the pulling forces of the muscles work for you and your swing.

A Primer on Movement

The following lists the ways muscle creates motion and enables your body to move.

- **Abduction:** Body segments moving away from center

- **Adduction:** Body segments moving toward center

- **Circumduction:** Rotation of body part in sequential movement

- **Extension:** Increase in angle between two body parts

- **Flexion:** Decrease in angle between two body parts (e.g., the elbow, hand, etc.)

- **Eversion:** Pronation of foot

- **Inversion:** Supination of foot

- **Inward Rotation:** Toward the middle

- **Outward Rotation:** Away from the middle

- **Pronation:** Rotation of forearm or hands downward

- **Rotation:** Circular motion of body segment

- **Supination:** Rotation of forearm or hands upward

Think back to when you first developed your swing. In the beginning, your structure dominated the motion of your swing. But as you progressed and you practiced more and more, a change began taking place. That change would have taken place at the point where you had mastered, to some degree, your golf skills. Function then determined your body structure or shape. What does that mean? It simply means that the muscles which came into play when you first learned to swing were not developed, so your swing was determined by your existing structure and the natural pulling forces your untrained muscles possessed. As your skill developed, and you practiced over and over, you developed new muscle groups that pulled on the joints and connective tissue, gradually changing the muscle's tone, size, and strength. Thus you created your own unique golf structure that involved your whole body.

This unique structure is registered in your brain, which sets up a neuromuscular connection that is unique to you. Each and every muscle, nerve, tendon, and other soft tissue developed to accommodate your skill. To change this with incorrect exercise will destroy all your hard work. This is why we do not recommend a specialized golf workout. Athletic trainers and exercise manuals that encourage such programs simply do not have a realistic point of view. They've missed the whole concept. We believe, and have witnessed time after time, the value of a total body workout, designed to maintain your unique musculature, without compromising your skill.

While there are many exercise routines that claim to be effective in building athletic fitness, the fact that so many exist and that trainers keep switching indicates how worthless they are. Only a routine that has passed the test of time can become the standard. The following are examples of some of the worthless routines being performed today:

- **The "Push-Pull" Method.** This implies that some muscles push and some muscles pull. This routine is adapted to supply exercises to be done on "push" days alternating with "pull" days. The only problem with this philosophy is simply that there are no "push" muscles. All muscles pull via a joint attached to an opposing bone and only give the appearance of pushing, thus rendering this routine useless. That's right—no skeletal muscles push, they only pull.

- **The "One-Body-Part" a Day Method.** This routine is popular with the very lazy. Its premise is that you train one muscle group (say, the chest muscles) one day, back muscles the next, and so on, until all the body parts are done. Then you start over again. The problem is that by the time you get back to the original body part, it has already atrophied because it has not received the adequate stimulation and circulation necessary for change.

- **Split Routine Method.** This involves working two or more body parts a day. For instance, exercising the chest, back, and shoulder muscles one day, and the arm, leg, and abdominal muscles the next. This is a very good bodybuilding type routine; unfortunately, it doesn't contribute to the balanced type of routine needed for athletes.

The human body is built as a unit. You take all of you wherever you go. When you eat, you feed all of you, and when you sleep, all of you sleeps. Get the point? Evidence supports that you should exercise it together. All the muscles interrelate and are tied together to form a sheath surrounding us. We advocate a total body workout, which involves training all of the major muscle groups together, in the same workout session.

Weight Lifting versus Lifting Weights: The Difference

There are people who *lift weights,* and there are those who *weight lift.* People who lift weights rely on the exercise apparatus for their result. Those who weight lift rely on the muscular contraction to move the given resistance, thus causing a more positive and targeted result. Those who lift weights are the effect of the exercise and not the effect of the result. Those who weight lift are causatively exercising, which, in a layperson's terms, means that the individual is getting more out of themselves and able to direct their mental concentration into each movement rather than relying on the machine to get the result. Achieving this higher state of awareness leads to more control. You quickly learn, when first exercising, that you have little control over specific muscle groups. However, with some practice, you will be able to isolate certain muscle groups and gain total control over them. The same can be said for golf. Although the golf club hits the ball, it is really the action guidance and stability of the muscle that creates the impact with the ball.

To be the effect of anything, whether it is exercise, life, or golf, means that you are not in control of the situation, but rather that some outside influence is affecting your results. Being causative, on the other hand, means that you are putting all of your energies and concentration into the present to create a result—which is the perfect swing. You are doing the exercise! The weights or machines are only tools to be used to increase the intensity and resistance. Never rely on the apparatus to do the exercise for you. You must do it!

Are the benefits of weight training for golf worth the price? *Yes!* For an individual interested in golf, no price can be paid to equal the value of true data. Beware, however, because the benefits of what is currently promoted as exercise are simply not worth it and may even be damaging to you! In our carefully considered opinion, most currently accepted methods of exercise will never actually produce anything in the way of lasting results simply because many of them are ill-conceived or delivered with bias, which is a far more pitiful commentary on the current state of affairs encompassing the field of exercise, fitness, and golf conditioning.

Exercise Considerations

In any sport, if you want to increase your skill, strength, or inherited ability, you need to challenge yourself to go beyond your current levels of achievement, or what is already easy for you. You cannot increase your overall physical power by merely repeating what is already easy. As we've said, the actual amount of exercise is meaningless unless the intensity of the work is high. You must consistently make an attempt at the "momentarily impossible" in all exercises. This means you exercise until it is impossible to move the resistance. Below a certain level of intensity, no amount of exercise will produce enough stimulation to create positive change. On the other hand, you must not train to the point that your body cannot recover. It's really very simple: work as hard as you can, for as brief a period as possible.

How often should you weight train? Supportive evidence suggests that you must work out three times per week, with very brief but intense exercise. This will produce full-sport conditioning benefits. Intense total-body workouts, where maximum effort is applied in an abbreviated period of time, produce extraordinary results, achieving approximately a 10:1 ratio over conventional exercise routines. It has been our experience, and it is an established fact, that strength, stability, and torque occur most effectively in muscle when exercise is performed intensely.

At what speed should you exercise? All routines should be performed at varying speeds. At the beginning of every repetition (rep) of an exercise, you should move slowly. As the set progresses, you should try to speed up the movement, never jerking on the way up or on the way down. Move in a steady, constant motion. For example, a number of reps should be selected—let's say eight (this doesn't mean that if you can do more, you shouldn't). Complete as many reps as possible in good form and then a couple more in not-so-good form, stopping only when additional movements become impossible. If the number of reps performed in good form is less than the target number, use the same amount of resistance the next workout as well. However, if you can perform the allotted number of reps in good form (in this case, eight), then the resistance should be increased for the next workout. If you constantly strive to increase the resistance and decrease exercise time, you'll find yourself capable of some amazing results, notably more explosive power and endurance.

Training with intensity is the basic principle involved in any form of worthwhile physical training. It is perfectly clear this type of training works, and it is equally clear that no other presently existing style of training is capable of producing such astonishing results so quickly. We have speculated for years that this type of training affects the survival of the muscle cells themselves, and that when pushed to their max, they change in fear of perishing.

If you're not willing to perform high-intensity exercises, then you will never produce the best results. Let's face it, nothing on this earth worth fighting for is easy, which is why we have leaders and champions so few in numbers. Only exercise routines that produce nothing short of muscle exhaustion will have the most positive effect for golfers. Ultimately, the increase in strength, stamina, and muscle stability depends on the recruitment of progenitor cells into muscle cells. High-intensity exercise, along with proper nutrition (discussed in Chapters 8 and 9), will facilitate this. The harder you train, the more force you put on a muscle during exercise, activating these progenitor cells that then create the muscle mass.

REST AND RECOVERY

Most people interested in sports conditioning either do too little or too much exercise. They fall into a rut, never recognizing that intensity training is better. In fact, the harder you train, the less time it should take. This brings us to the third leg on our conditioning routine: recovery.

The body responds well to intense exercise and recovers easily. It does poorly when even a poor level of exercise is done for too long a period of time. You can only *over*train when you work *over*time.

When you have worked the muscle to failure with an intense, strict, little-rest style of training (see exercises in the next chapter), the muscles and related systems need twenty-four hours to recover, sometimes more in the beginning. The body makes certain demands for materials required for conditioning. The primary limiting factor in creating the ultimate body for golf via exercise is the ability of the body's systems to make the chemical changes necessary to repair itself within an allotted time period. If you work out too soon after your last exercise session, then little or nothing in the way of conditioning and fitness can occur.

Hard Work Induces Change—
Time Permits that Change to Take Place

Within the human system, there exist a number of regulatory subsystems whose functions aid conditioning and recovery. Respiration, digestion, sleep, and the endocrine system are several examples. We have, in previous chapters, tried to bring their purposes and functions to your attention so you would have a better-than-average working knowledge of how exercise and recovery affect your Atomic Golf goals.

Recovery is simply a matter of supply and demand. If the supply is not available to aid recovery, the body will reduce its ability to demand. The body needs building materials, which consist of protein, carbohydrates, fats, and oxygen. The body demands sugar for energy, proteins for rebuilding, and vitamins and minerals to carry this out. It is immensely important for you to understand that intense exertion is required to induce physical change. Low intensity (remember, intensity is the most amount of work possible in the shortest possible time) produces low results, if any. Smart, hard work is required. Your recovery ability is limited, so keep those workouts fast, hard, and brief, with one or two days in between to rest and recover.

A failure to understand these properties of exercise has led to the present debacle in exercise circles, especially in golf. Trainers work their clients

Helpful Hints for a Successful Workout

- Limit your weekly workouts to three training sessions for the entire body, including the legs.

- Limit the length of your workouts to no more than forty-five minutes.

- Seldom perform more than three sets of any one exercise—and never perform more than five sets of any one exercise.

- Make unceasing efforts to progress. Always attempt to produce at least some sign of progress in every set of every exercise (by doing the set faster, with heavier resistance, etc.).

- Pay particular attention to the "form" of your exercises. Do not permit the style of performance to degenerate into a mere "going through the motions."

- In general, select the "hardest" exercises—which we do in Chapter 11—and perform them in the most difficult manner possible. If a particular style of performance makes an exercise easier, it is most assuredly less productive.

too much, never too hard. What matters is the intensity with which you work, following the guidelines of the routine, in the shortest period possible. Quick in/quick out builds a better body throughout!

Intensity training is beneficial to our program because it sharply reduces training time. Our use of "cycle training" encourages this. Cycle training involves doing one exercise after another with little or no rest until the routine is done. It should be clearly understood, however, that we are *not* using cycle training merely in an attempt to save training time. We are using it because it is an absolute requirement for producing the best possible results, and it is a requirement because of the extremely short initial recovery times encountered in muscular activity. In order to work a particular muscle as hard as it must be worked to induce maximum conditioning—while staying within the limits imposed by the overall recovery ability of the system—you must use cycle-type training routines. When this is done properly, only a few, very brief cycles are required, or even desired.

- *Never* terminate a particular set simply because you have completed a certain number of repetitions. A set is properly finished only when additional movement is utterly impossible. Curl until you can't even begin to bend your arms. Squat until you can't start up from the low position. Press until you cannot move the bar away from your shoulders or chest.

- If you can perform your "guide number" of repetitions, or *more*, then that is your signal to increase the resistance in that particular exercise at your next workout.

- An advanced trainee does not need "more" exercise than a beginner; they simply need "harder" exercise in a shorter period of time. An advanced trainee may be able to endure more exercise, but it is not a requirement and will almost always lead to a situation where additional progress comes to a halt or slows to a snail's pace if the increased amount of exercise is not met with a fast pace.

- Judge your progress by measurable increases in strength. When you can perform the same number of repetitions with twice as much resistance, then your muscles will be at least twice as conditioned as they were at the start, and probably twice as toned.

Doing more cycles may or may not induce more growth stimulation. Check out the exercises in Chapter 11 for more information.

Note: Cycle-type training does from time to time involve using a treadmill or stationary bicycle.

WHERE AND WHEN TO BEGIN

In any exercise program, there are guidelines to follow. The suggestions below are scientifically based and contain sound guidelines that should be followed when starting the conditioning routines provided in Chapter 11:

1. Before starting an exercise program, check your general health with a physician.

2. Keep records of your progress in weight and measurements. Take pictures of yourself, if possible.

3. Note any previous injuries you have or may have had.

4. Exercise on a gradient level, a little at a time, building up to high intensity.

5. Stay focused. Always keep your goals and purposes in front of you.

6. In conditioning training, always do a total body workout, working the largest muscles first (see Chapter 11).

7. Never exercise with heavy weights. It is best to increase the intensity instead.

8. Eliminate bad health habits such as smoking, drinking, and inadequate sleep.

9. Exercise consistently in a pleasant atmosphere.

10. Challenge yourself.

It has been obvious for decades that exercise is capable of producing a level of strength and clarity of mind far beyond mortal levels. The earliest archeological finds depict pictures of people exercising. Obviously, even back then, people understood there was a way to achieve greatness far beyond what they were born with. Today, men and women strive to reach unheard-of levels in every endeavor of their lives. Our goal is simply to educate you in ways and methods that can bring about such dynamic changes in your golf game that you'll never be the same again.

Atomic Conditioning Routines

11

*I*n this chapter, we bring you the most tried-and-true conditioning routines that have been shown to bring about exceptional results quickly. The following is a list of the terms and basic equipment you will need to know in order to follow the exercise routines in this chapter and when working out in a gym setting:

- Ankle weights—adjustable weighted straps that attach to the ankle

- Barbell—a single bar held with both hands to do an exercise

- Decline bench—an adjustable bench designed to be angled down so that the head is positioned lower than the legs

- Dumbbells—a small weight that is held in each hand; they are available in various poundages

- Exercise machine—any one of the various number of exercise machines designed specifically for each body part

- Flat bench—an exercise bench that is used for any exercise requiring a flat surface

- Frequency of exercise—how often exercise is engaged in on a weekly basis

- Full/half repetitions—any exercise consisting of a full movement followed by half a movement, and counted as one rep

- Half/full repetitions—any exercise consisting of half a movement followed by a full movement, and counted as one rep

- Incline bench—an adjustable bench designed to be raised to different angles for different exercises

- Intensity of exercise—most amount of work that can be done in the shortest amount of time

- Pulley machine—machine used for various applications by use of a system of cables and pulleys

- Recovery—adequate time must be allotted between one workout and the next in order to gain maximum results

- Repetitions (reps)—number of movements performed of a single exercise

- Resistance—amount of weight moved that can be performed through its full range of motion

- Rest—period taken between sets; as little rest as possible is recommended

- Seated bench—chair-like bench used to perform seated exercises

- Sets—number of groups of repetitions performed; a brief rest is required between sets

- Static hold—any exercise done with a full repetition and held motionless halfway down

- Super sets—any two exercises done in succession with no rest between

CONDITIONING ROUTINES AND GUIDELINES

The Atomic Golf Exercise Program is divided into three levels. We recommend that everyone begin at Level I. Unless a golfer's general fitness level is excellent, he or she will achieve less than their optimum level of play. Levels I and II are aimed at conditioning the body and building a solid physical foundation for the real work to follow, or the exercises needed to create the true Atomic Golfer. Each level builds on the last. Each level is designed to accommodate the next level. It is necessary to do this in order to prevent injury and overworking. The conditioning exercises in Levels I and II are also cardio in nature.

Level I: Preparatory Training
- Beginning Routine I
- Beginning Routine II

Level II: Intermediate Training
- Intermediate Routine I

- Intermediate Routine II
- Intermediate Routine III

Level III: Strength Training
- Advanced Routine
- Advanced Routine II
- Advanced Strength Routine
- Advanced Explosive Power Routine
- Advanced Power Endurance Routine (with aerobic component)

In the early levels (Levels I and II), we recommend that 50 percent of your time be spent practicing your skill (golfing), and the other 50 percent be spent conditioning your body's joints, muscles, ligaments, and support structure, with attention devoted to injured or weak areas. At this point, the volume of exercise is more important than the amount of time you spend exercising. Emphasis in the workout is placed on a large variety of exercises and different joint movements.

In Level I, most of the exercises are to be done with dumbbells and ankle weights to help develop joints and stabilizer muscles (muscles that reinforce the skeletal structure and bone to keep you steady and focused). As you progress to the intermediate routines in Level II, barbells and exercise machines will be added. Do not increase the weight unless specified. Further down the road, in the advanced routines in Level III, you will add strength-training exercise with resistance machines to prevent injury and strain.

In general, your preparatory training in Level I should not last more than three months. In Level II, your generalized conditioning continues and a more intense training period begins. With each level, the volume of exercise increases with a corresponding decrease in exercise time. This will increase the intensity and the difficulty of the exercises. The routines are fairly demanding, but the results are colossal. Without the proper completion of Level I, however, the golfer-in-training will not be able to successfully move on to Level II and above. Be careful to never go on to another level until you have successfully completed the level before it.

When performing the exercise routines outlined above, it is important to follow these guidelines:

- Wear lightweight, loose-fitting clothes and have a water bottle handy.

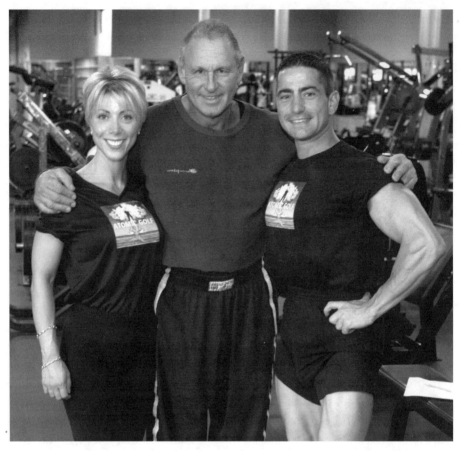

The Atomic Golf team: From left, Darlene Iaquinta, Steve Michalik, and Michael Manavian.

- Perform each rep slowly at first, using a full range of motion, then gradually increase the speed.

- Breathe normally and rhythmically. Do not hold your breath continuously for several consecutive repetitions. Try to develop a rhythmic pattern of breathing that corresponds to the exercise cycle.

- Write down your exercises in a logbook, recording the poundage as well as how hard or easy that resistance was.

- Write down how long your workout took from start to finish.

  Note: Before beginning this, or any exercise regimen, it is important to consult your physician.

LEVEL I: PREPARATORY TRAINING

The following routines require the use of dumbbells and ankle weights. Pick a weight you can perform twenty-five repetitions with easily. Rest as long as it takes between exercises to normalize your breathing. Do this routine three times a week. Participate in some form of aerobic activity at least two days a week for at least thirty minutes per session. This general preparatory training period should not last more than three months, after which you should have attained a good level of physical conditioning.

Beginning Routine I

Begin with a single set of twenty-five reps for each exercise, and complete the entire routine. This is one cycle. Work quickly, but maintain form. When completing one set of twenty-five reps becomes relatively easy, advance to two sets of twenty-five for each exercise. Eventually, work your way up to four sets of twenty-five for each exercise. When you're able to complete this final cycle, you're ready to move on to Beginning Routine II.

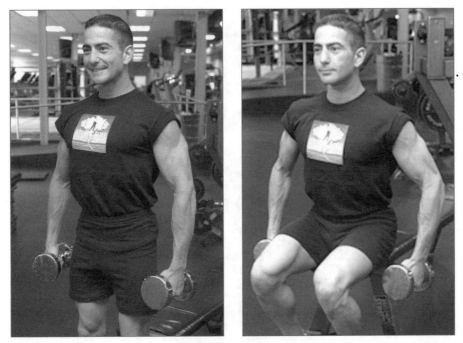

Bench squat: Upper legs and hips

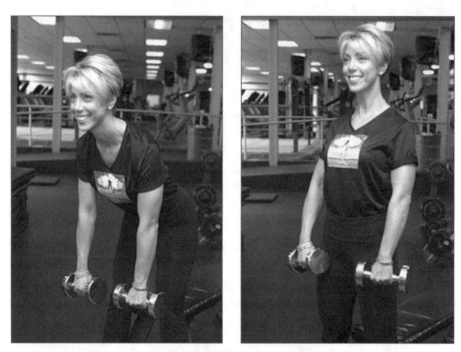

Partial dead lifts: Legs and hips

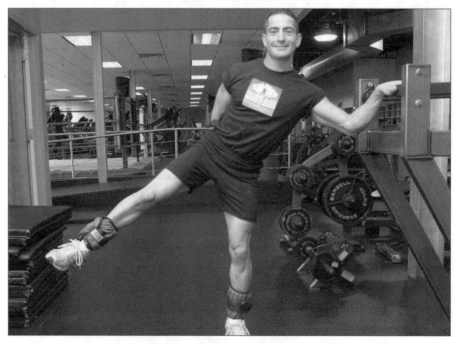

Side leg lifts (with ankle weights): Hips

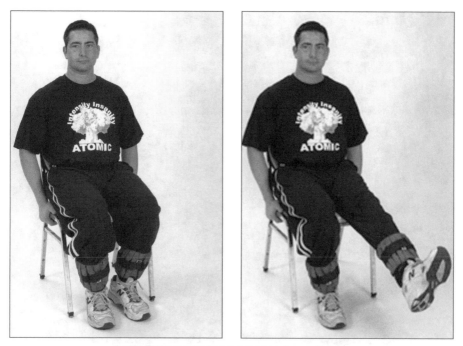

Seated alternate leg extension: Lower thighs

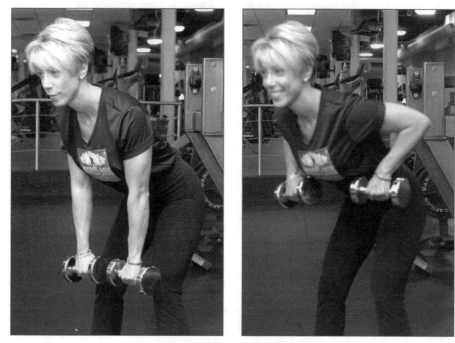

Bent-over dumbbell row: Back

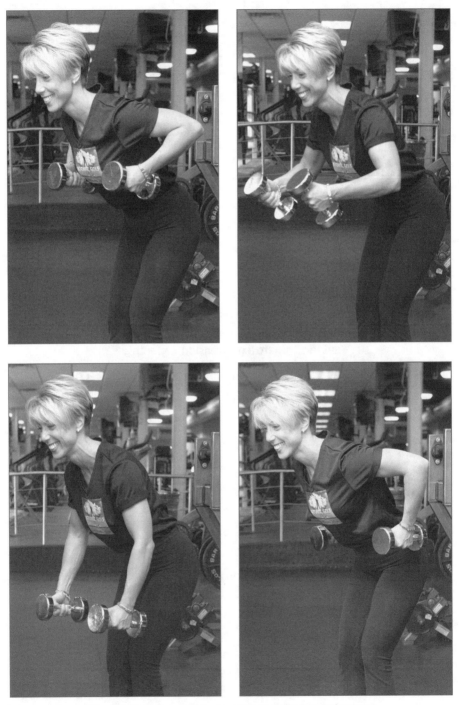

Churns: Back *(sequence goes left to right, top to bottom)*

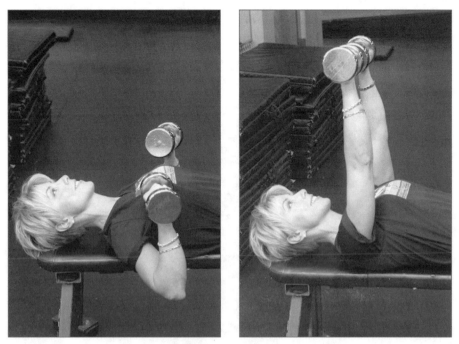

Lying chest press: Chest

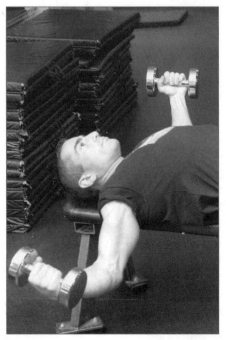
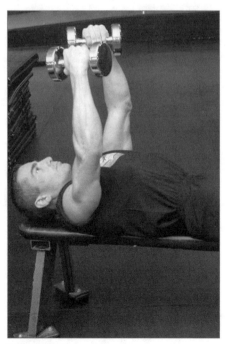

Lying dumbbell flies: Chest

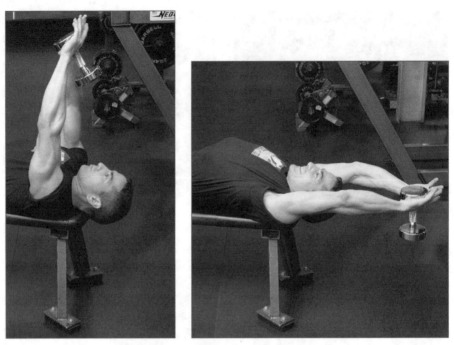

Lying dumbbell pullovers: Structure

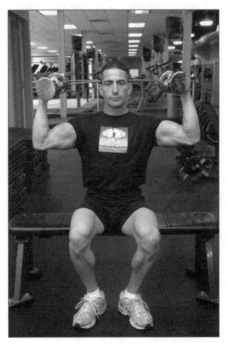 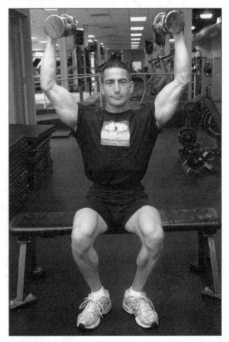

Seated dumbbell press: Shoulders

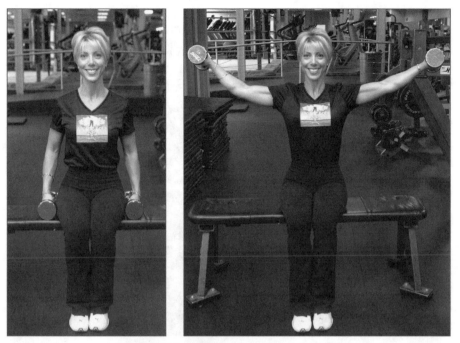

Seated side dumbbell laterals: Shoulders

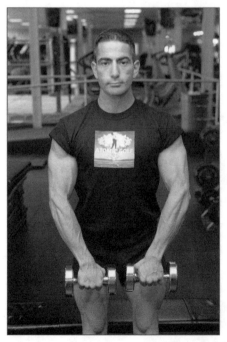 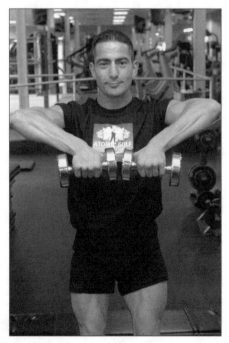

Standing upright row: Shoulders

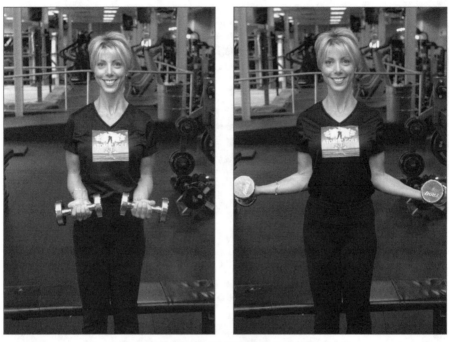

Standing dumbbell rotators: Upper back

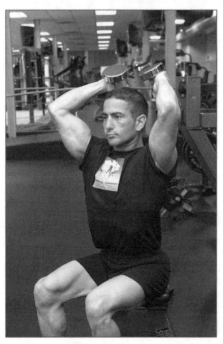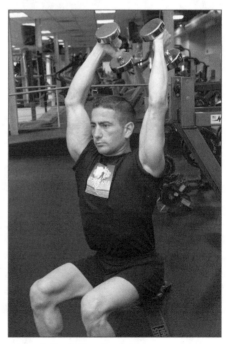

Overhead tricep extension: Arms (triceps)

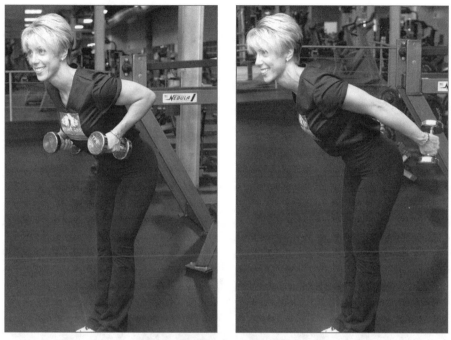

Tricep kickbacks: Arms (triceps)

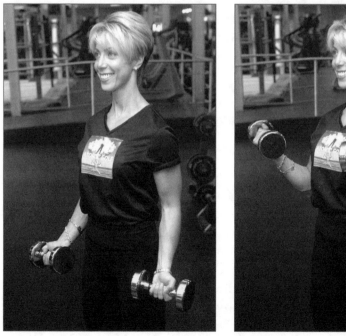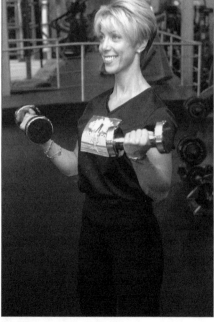

Dumbbell curls (with palms facing up): Arms (biceps)

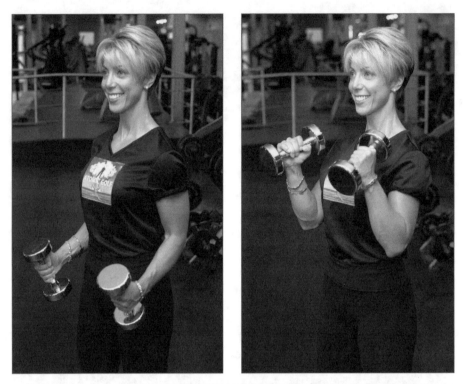

Zottman curls (with thumbs facing up and palms facing toward each other):
Arms (biceps)

Beginning Routine II

This is a super-set routine, meaning that two exercises are combined for each body part. They should be performed as if they were one exercise, with little to no resting period between techniques.

To begin, start with one set of fifteen reps for each exercise until the entire routine is complete. When this becomes relatively easy, advance to two sets of fifteen reps, and then three sets of fifteen reps. After you've mastered three sets of fifteen reps, advance to two sets of twenty-five reps. When you've mastered this final challenge, you're ready to advance to Level II.

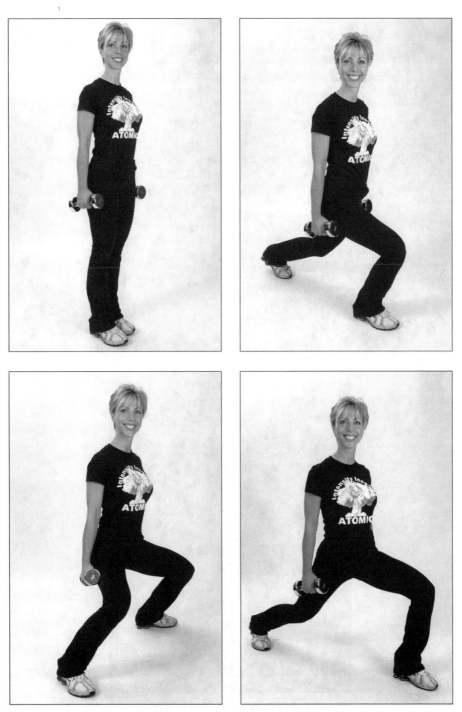

Three-way lunge: Upper legs and hips

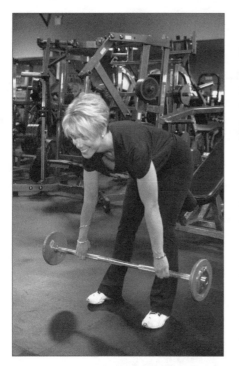
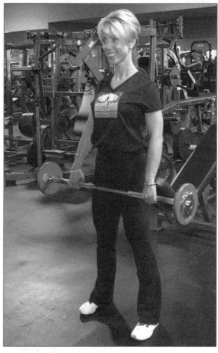

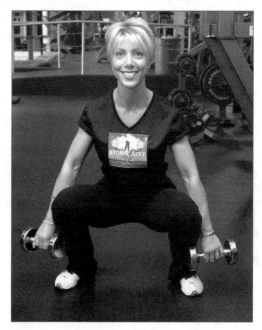

Dead lift with frog squat: Back of legs and hips

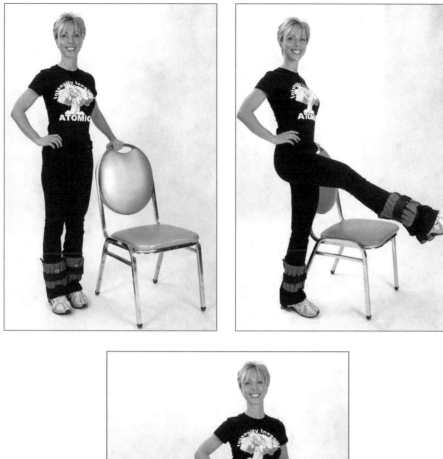

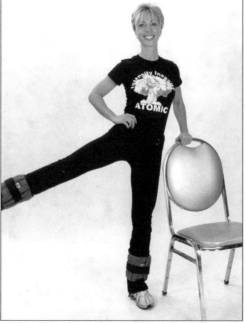

Front/side leg lifts: Butt and hips

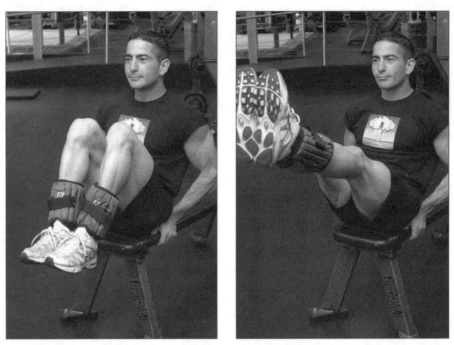

Knee-up and leg extensions (lift off ground, then kick out): Lower thighs

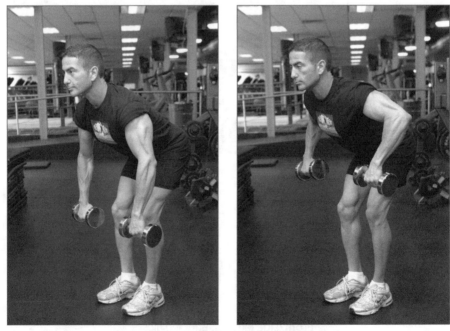

Bent-over dumbbell row with churns: Back

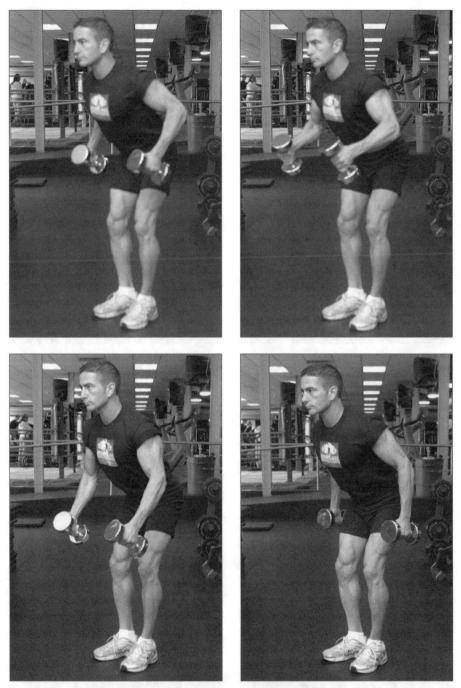

Bent-over dumbbell row with churns: Back
(sequence goes left to right, top to bottom)

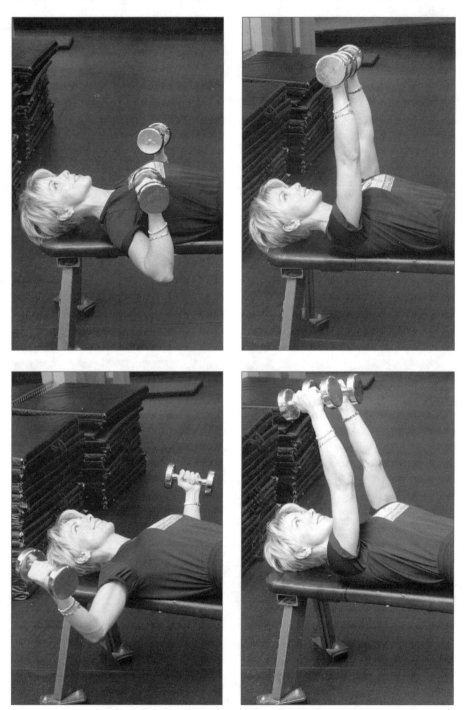

Lying chest press with lying dumbbell flies: Chest

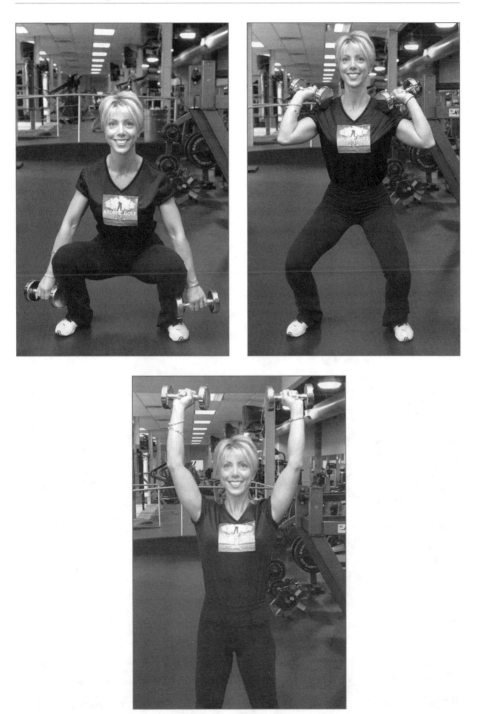

Standing dumbbell clean and press: Shoulders/trapezius muscle

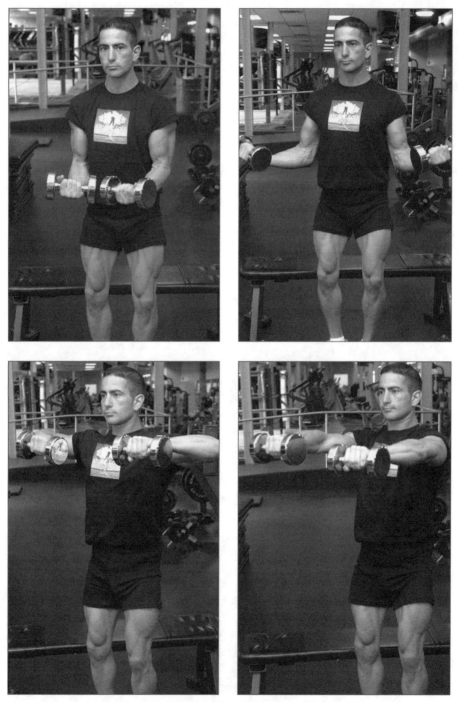

Standing dumbbell rotators and push-outs: Shoulders

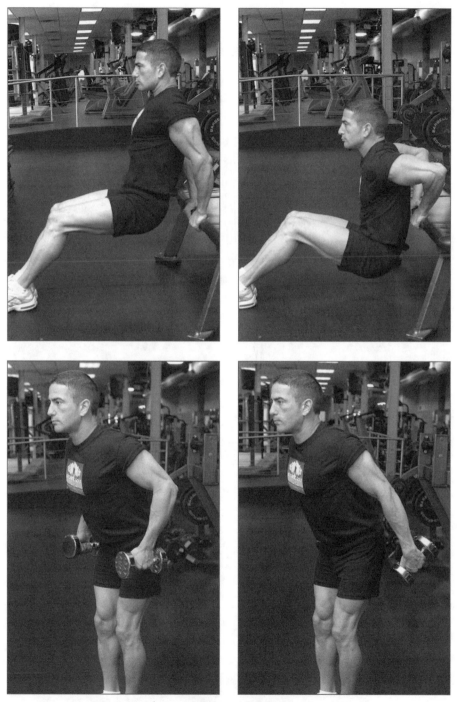

Bench/chair dips with tricep kickbacks: Arms (triceps)

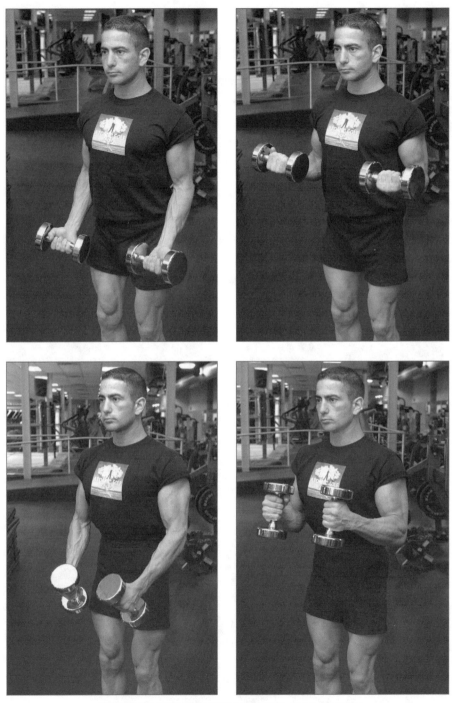

Dumbbell curls with Zottman curls: Arms (biceps)

LEVEL II: INTERMEDIATE TRAINING

These routines should not be attempted by anyone who has not mastered Beginning Routines I and II. These routines require the use of barbells, dumbbells, and exercise machinery found in most gyms, and they should be performed three times a week for one month. In these exercises, begin with a weight that is challenging. Continue with intense aerobic activity on nontraining days. Upon completion, our goal is that you will be in extremely good physical condition.

Intermediate Routine I

This is a simple, progressive routine. You will increase weight as you decrease repetitions. Do each exercise in perfect form. Only use the rush factor between sets and exercise—meaning there is little or no rest between sets.

To begin, do this routine one time through and time it. When you are able to successfully complete two full sets as hard and as fast as possible, while maintaining good form and decreasing time, you are ready to move on to Intermediate Routine II.

- First set: 15 reps (with a low resistance)

- Second set: 8 reps (with a higher resistance)

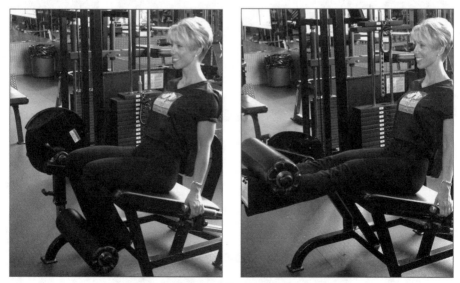

Leg extension machine: Legs, hips, and butt

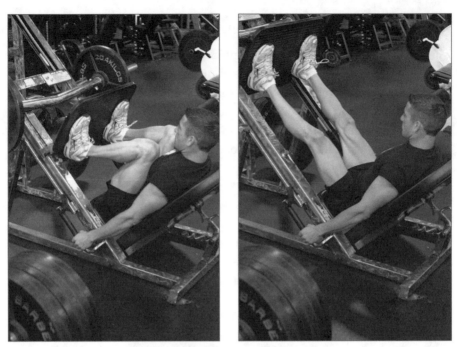

Leg press machine: Legs, hips, and butt

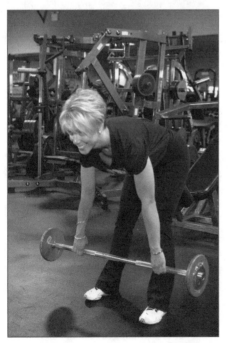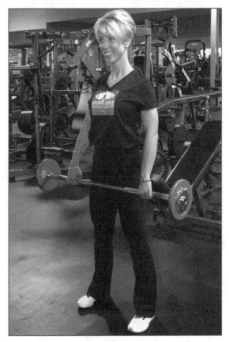

Dead lifts: Legs, hips, and butt

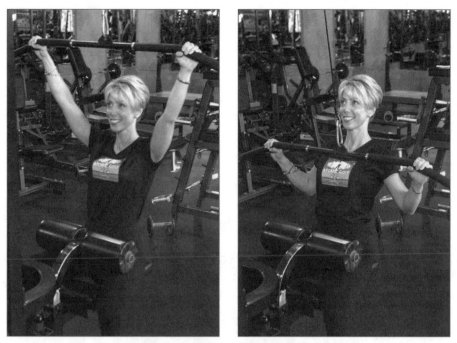

Pull-down to front on lateral machine: Back

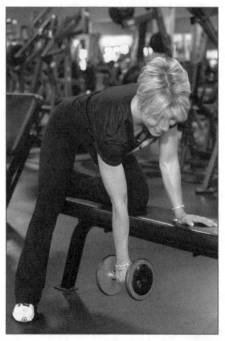 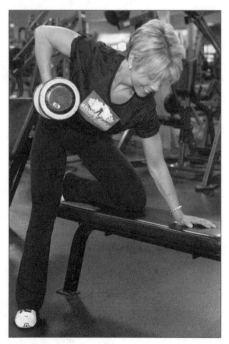

One-arm dumbbell row: Back

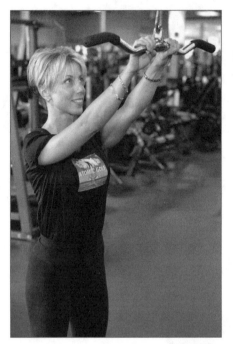 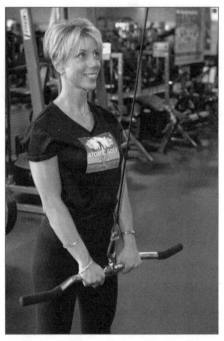

Straight-arm pulls: Back

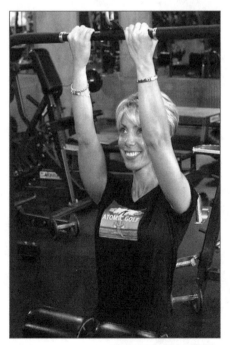 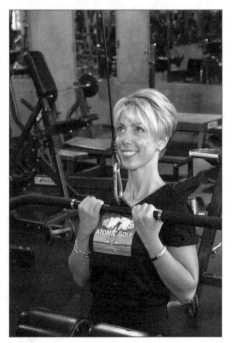

Reverse grip pull-downs on lat machine: Back

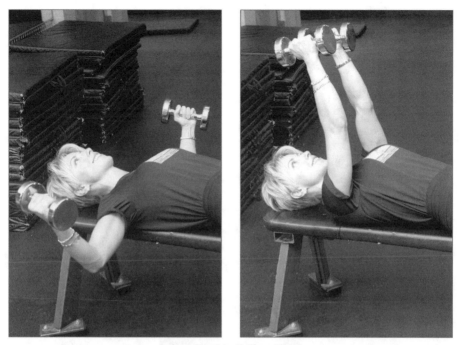

Lying dumbbell flies: Chest

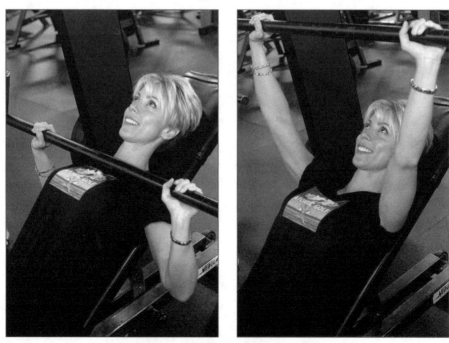

Incline bench press on Smith machine: Chest

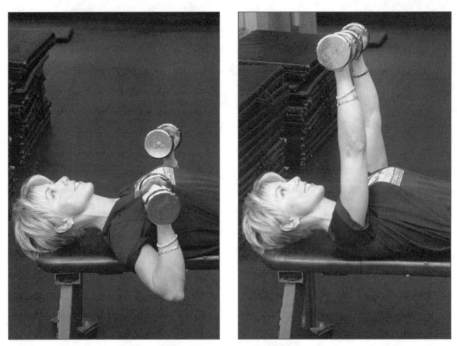

Lying chest press (with dumbbells): Chest

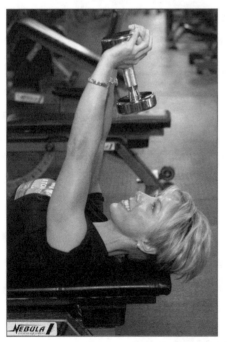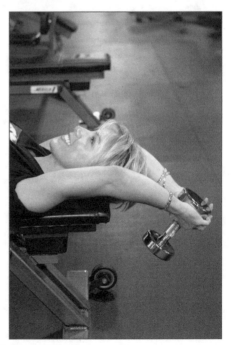

Dumbbell pullovers: Chest

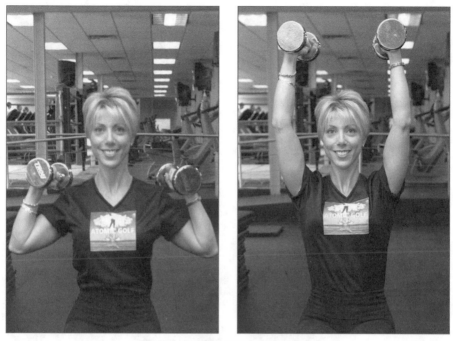

Seated dumbbell press: Shoulders

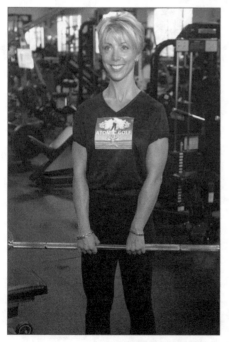
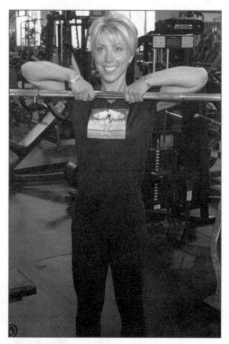

Standing upright row (with barbell): Shoulders

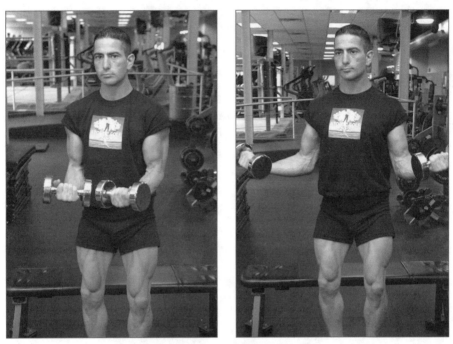

Standing dumbbell rotators: Shoulders

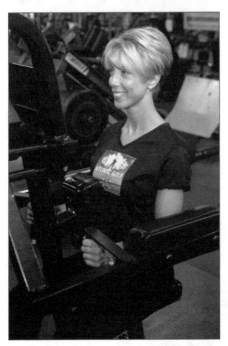
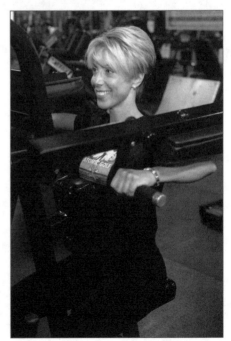

Lateral raise machine: Shoulders

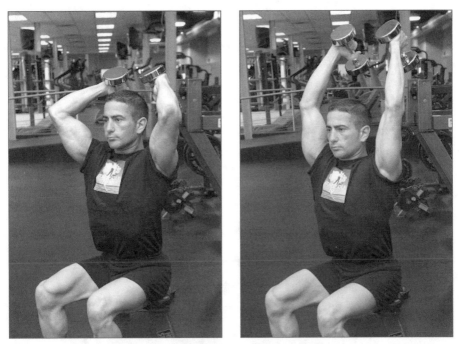

Overhead dumbbell tricep extension: Arms (triceps)

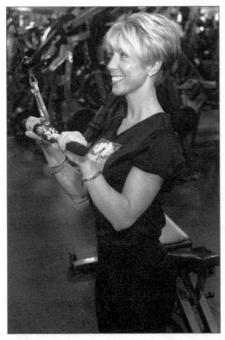 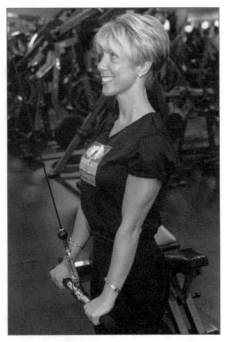

Tricep pushdowns: Arms (triceps)

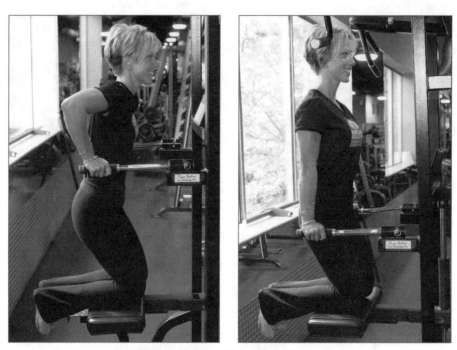

Dips on dip machine: Arms (triceps)

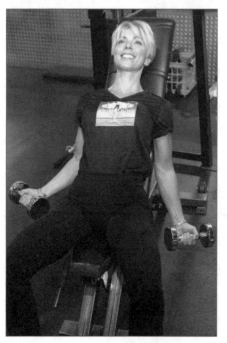
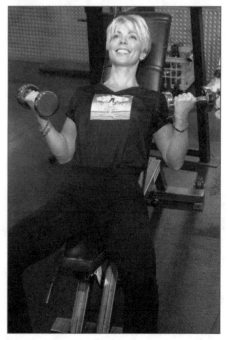

Incline bench dumbbell curls: Arms (biceps)

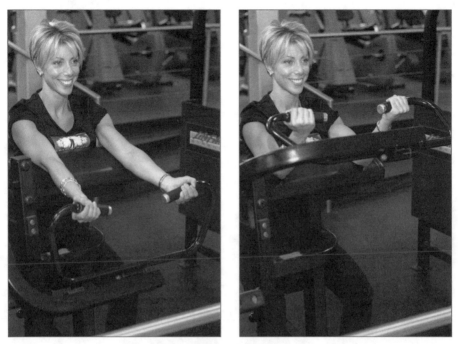

Curl machine: Arms (biceps)

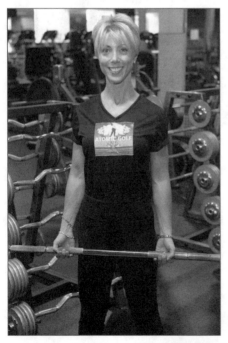
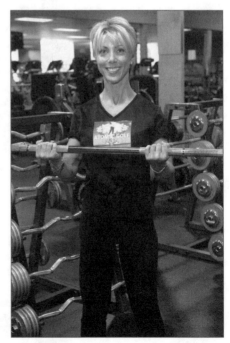

Barbell curl: Arms (biceps)

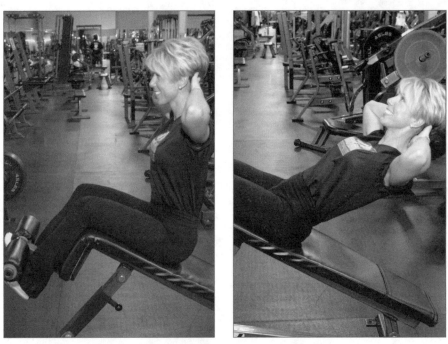

Roman chair sit-ups: Abdominals

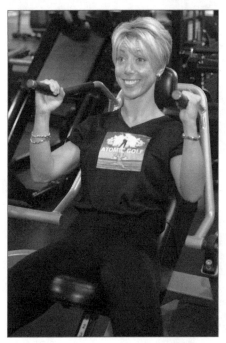
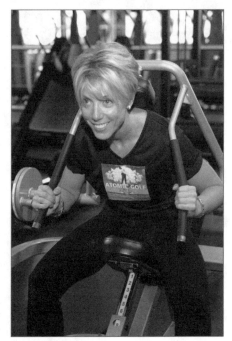

Abdominal machine: Abdominals

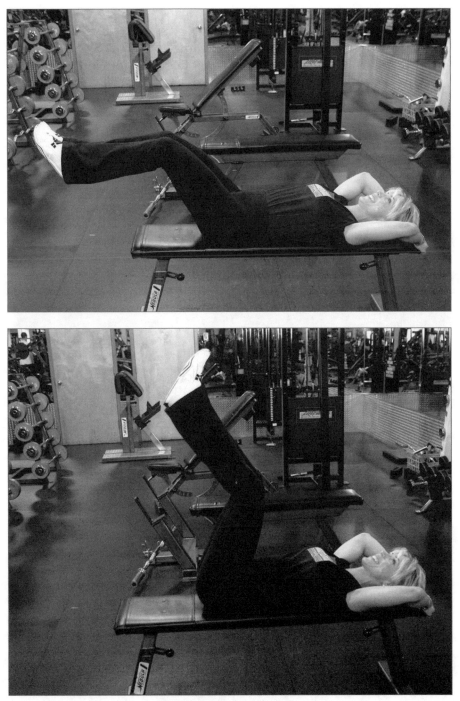

Lying leg raises: Abdominals

Intermediate Routine II

This is another progressive routine. Follow the pattern of repetitions described below until you have completed the entire routine. Increase the resistance with each set.

- First set: 25 reps (with a low resistance)
- Second set: 15 reps (with a higher resistance)
- Third set: 8 reps (with an even higher resistance)

After you are able to successfully complete this routine one time through, increase your effort to complete the pattern of three sets twice for each exercise until the entire routine is completed. When you are able to successfully complete the pattern three times for each exercise, you are ready to advance to Intermediate Routine III.

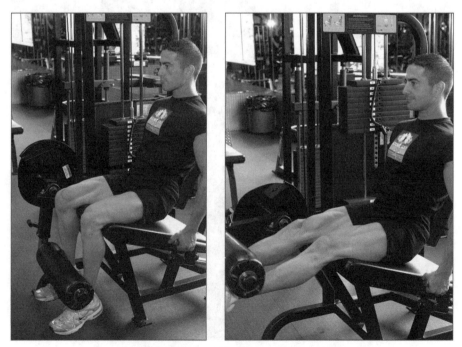

Leg extension machine: Legs, hips, and butt

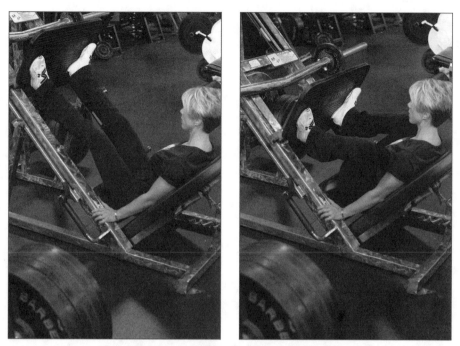

Leg press machine: Legs, hips, and butt

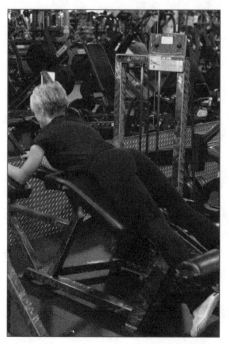
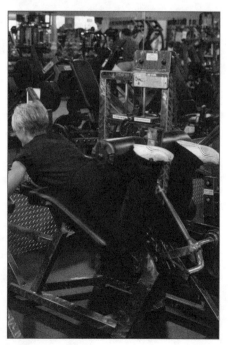

Leg curl machine: Legs, hips, and butt

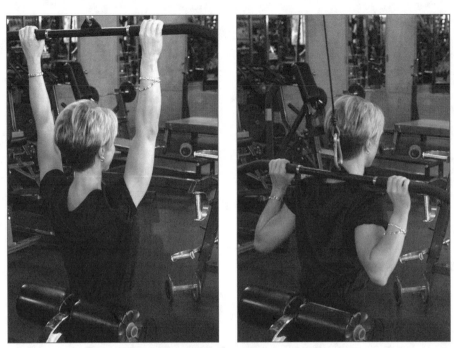

Rear lateral machine pull-downs: Back

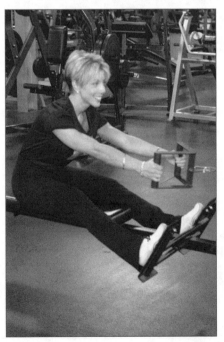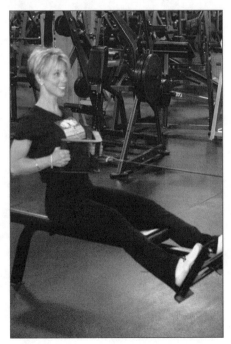

Seated cable row: Back

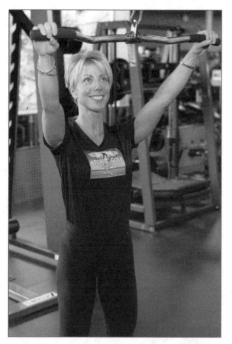
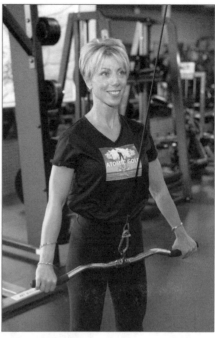

Straight-arm pulls: Back

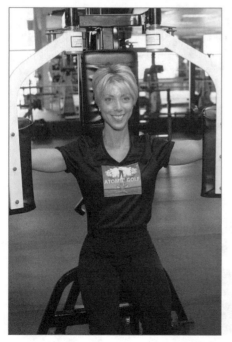
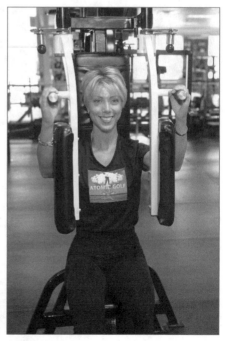

Peck deck machine: Chest

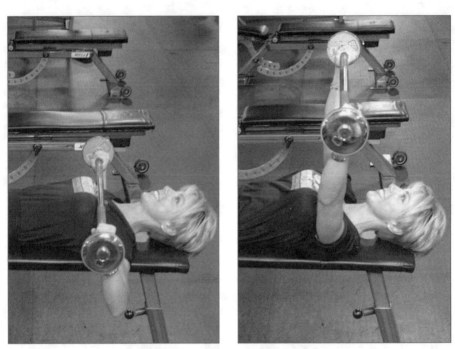

Bench press (barbell or machine): Chest

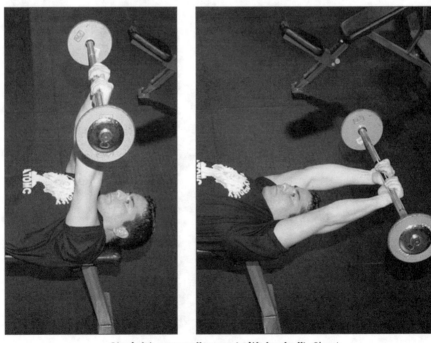

Straight-arm pullovers (with barbell): Chest

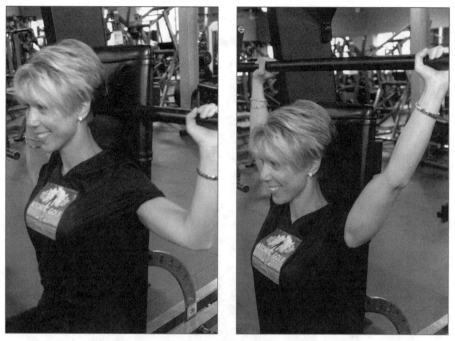

Press behind neck (barbell or machine): Shoulders

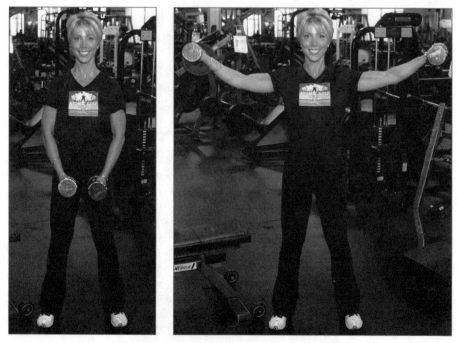

Lateral raises (machine or barbell): Shoulders

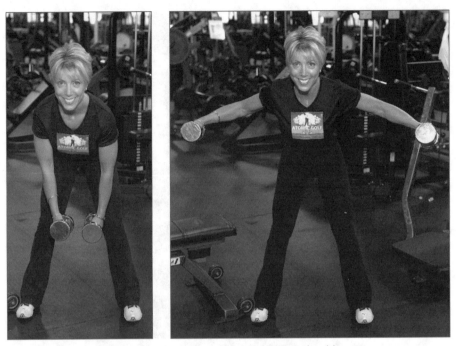

Bent-over laterals (with dumbbells): Shoulders

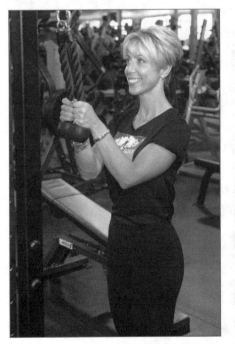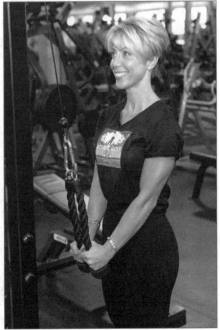

Tricep pushdowns: Arms (triceps)

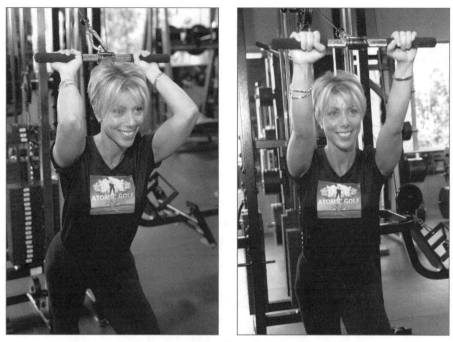

Tricep push-outs: Arms (triceps)

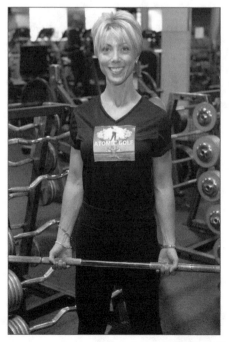
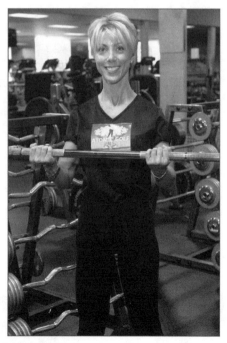

Barbell curls: Arms (biceps)

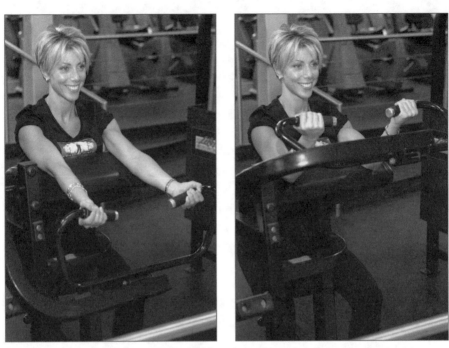

Curl machine: Arms (biceps)

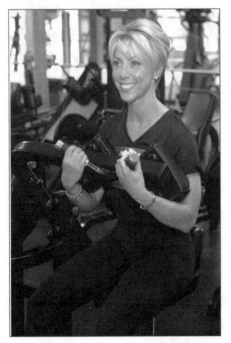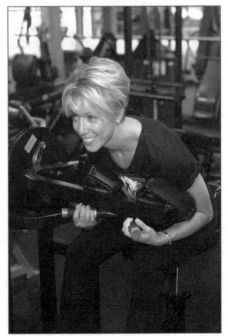

Abdominal machine: Abdominals

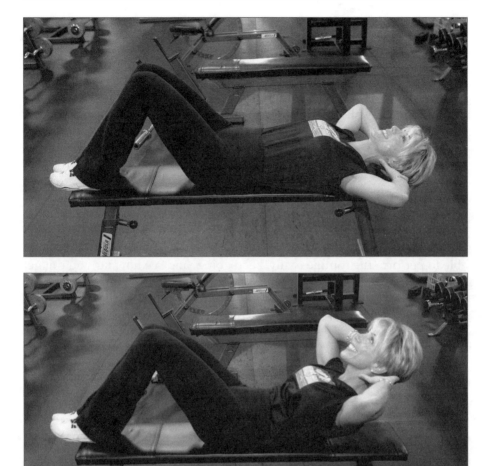

Lying crunch: Abdominals

Intermediate Routine III

Follow directions for Intermediate Routine II but with increased resistance.

LEVEL III: STRENGTH TRAINING

The routines in Level III should not be attempted by anyone who has not mastered Intermediate Routines I and II. These routines require the use of ankle weights, barbells, dumbbells, and exercise machinery found in most gyms. They should be performed three times a week for one month. Upon their completion, our goal is that you will be in exceptional physical condition!

Advanced Routine I

To start, follow the pattern of repetitions described below until you have completed the entire routine one time through, and time it. After you are able to perform the routine easily, keep going, and see how far you can get a second time. The goal is to increase the weight you can lift while decreasing the time it takes you to perform the entire set. When you have mastered this and are able to successfully complete the routine a third time, you are ready to move on to Advanced Routine II.

- First set: 15 reps (heaviest as possible for 15 reps, this may take some adjusting at first to know how heavy you can go)

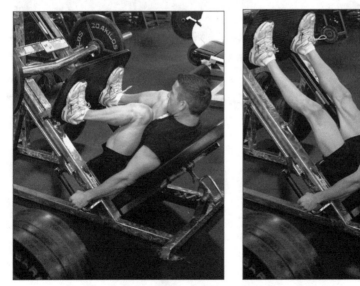

Leg press machine: Legs, hips, and butt

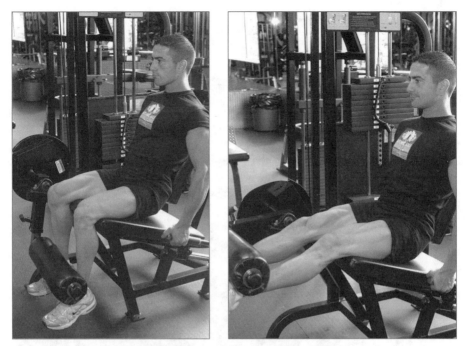

Leg extension machine: Legs, hips, and butt

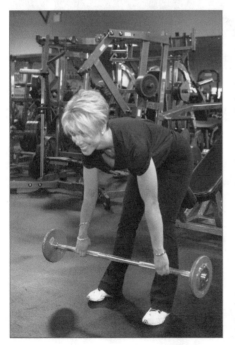
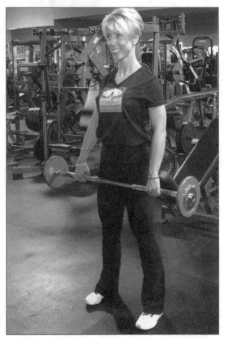

Dead lifts: Legs, hips, and butt

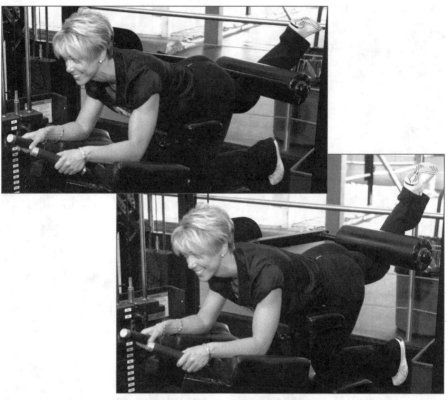

Hip machine: Legs, hips, and butt

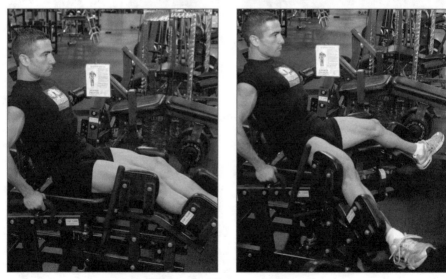

Outer thigh machine: Legs, hips, and butt

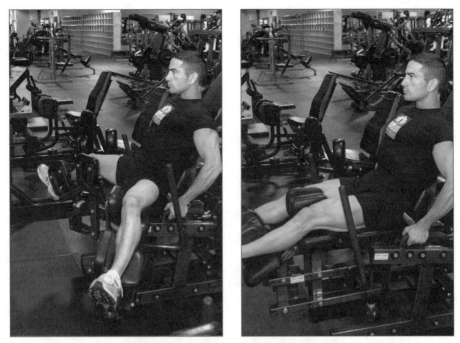

Inner thigh machine: Legs, hips, and butt

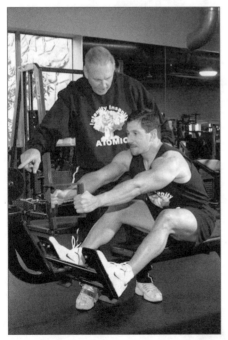
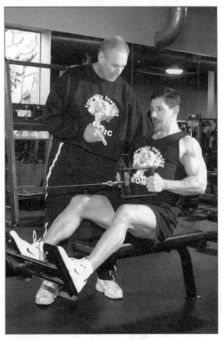

Seated row machine: Back

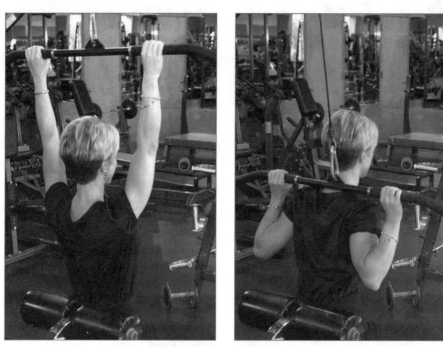

Pull-down behind neck: Back

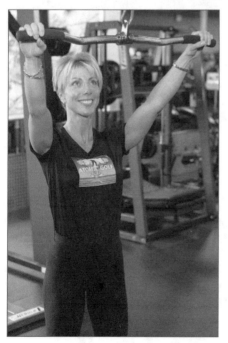
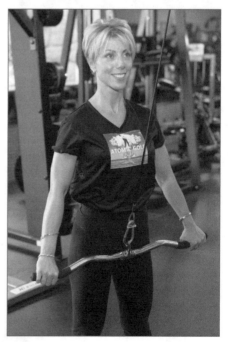

Straight-arm pulls: Back

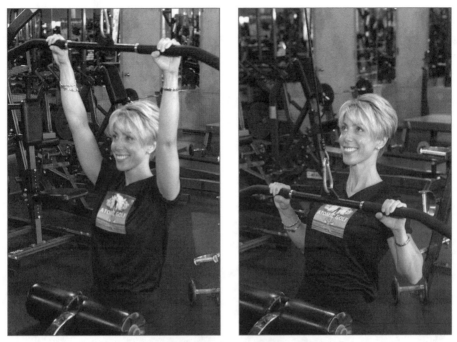

Close grip pull to front on lateral machine: Back

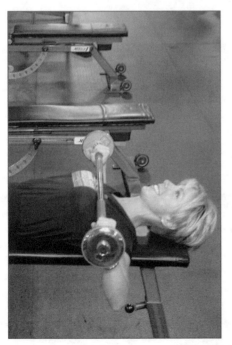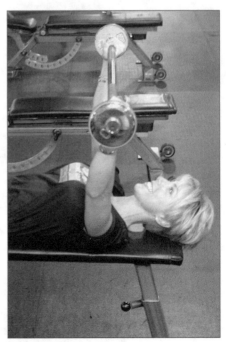

Bench press: Chest

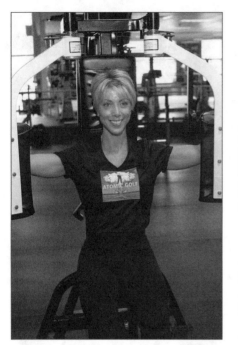 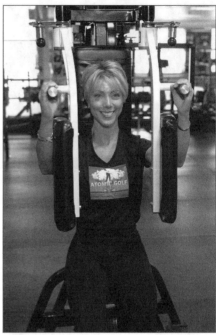

Peck deck: Chest

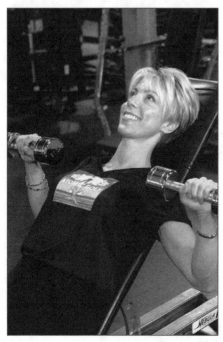 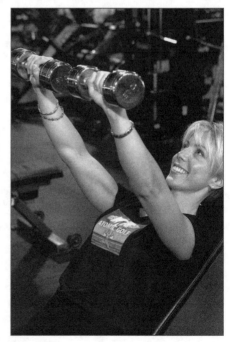

Incline dumbbell press: Chest

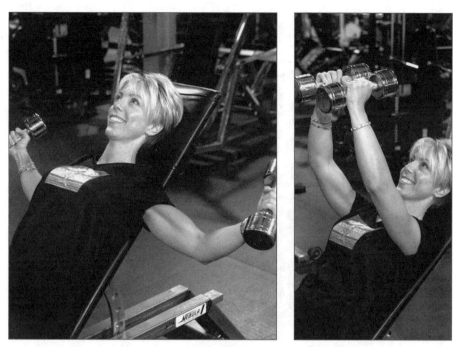

Incline flies: Chest

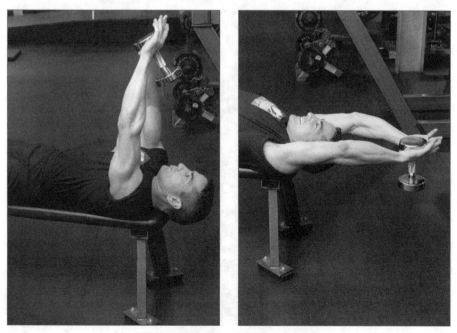

Lying dumbbell pullovers: Structure

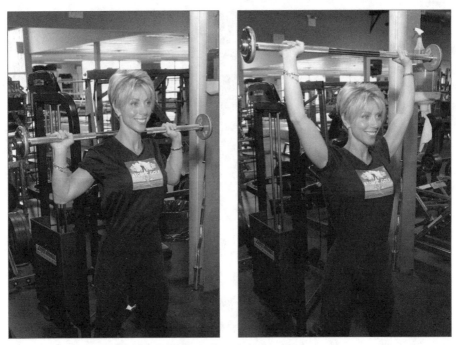

Behind-neck press: Shoulders

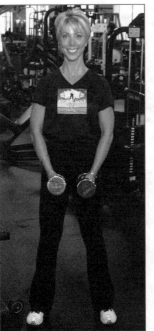
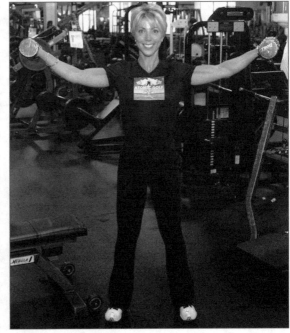

Side dumbbell lateral raise: Shoulders

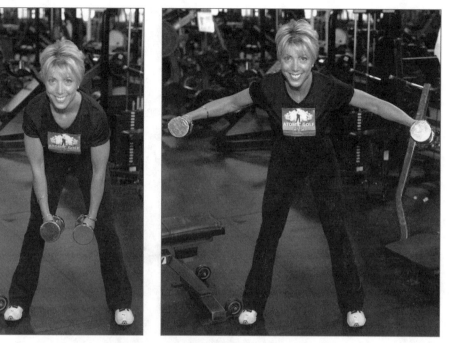

Bent-over dumbbell laterals: Shoulders

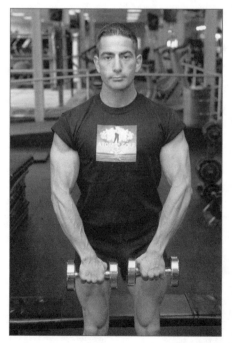
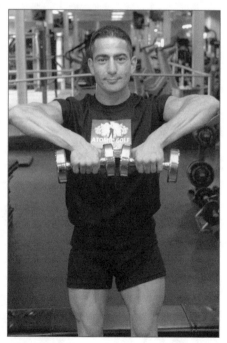

Upright rows: Shoulders

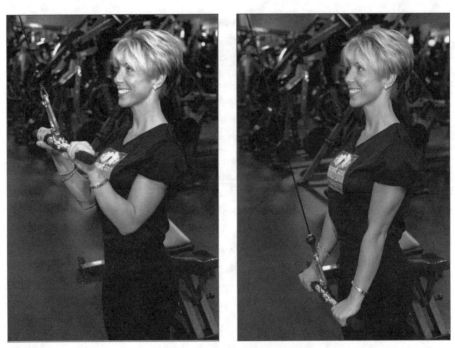

Tricep pushdowns: Arms (triceps)

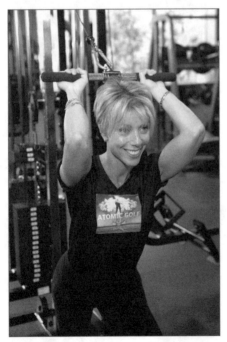
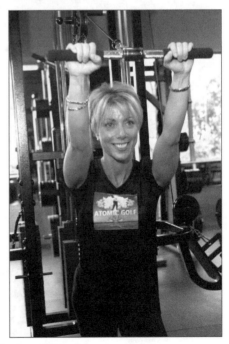

Tricep push-outs: Arms (triceps)

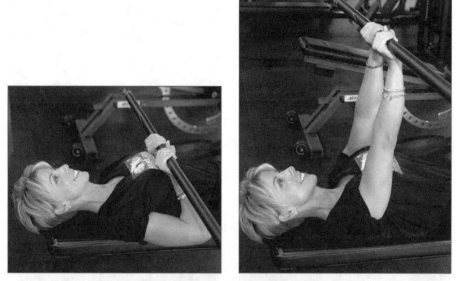

Close grip bench press with barbell: Arms (triceps)

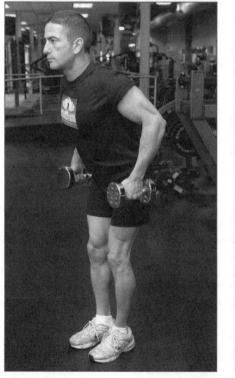
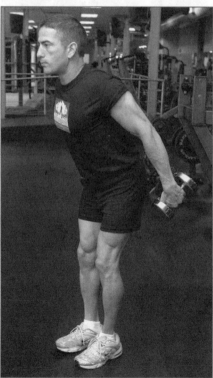

Dumbbell kickbacks: Arms (triceps)

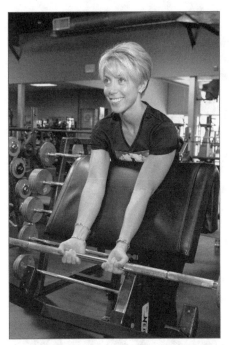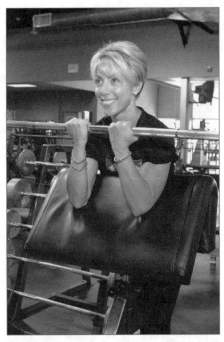

Barbell curl: Arms (biceps)

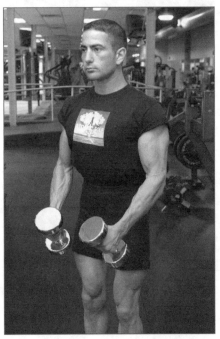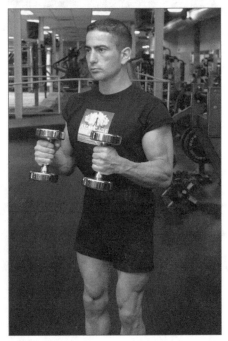

Dumbbell hammer curl: Arms (biceps)

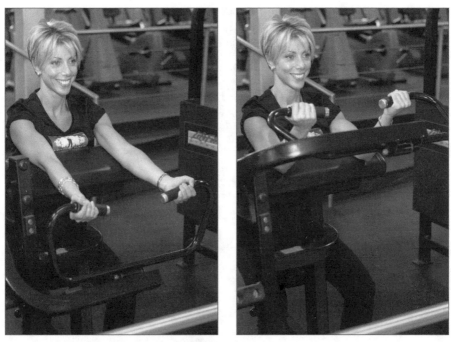

Curl machine: Arms (biceps)

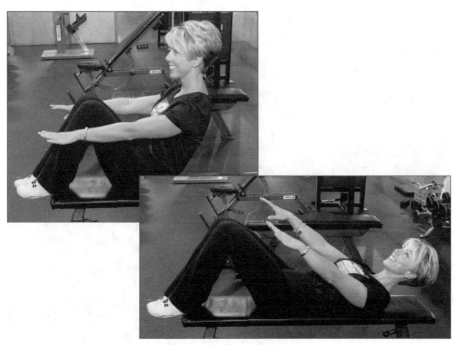

Crunch on bench: Abdominals

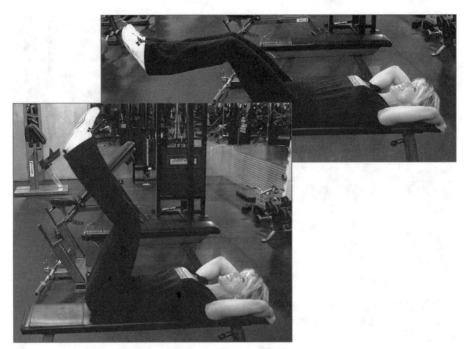

Lying leg raises: Abdominals

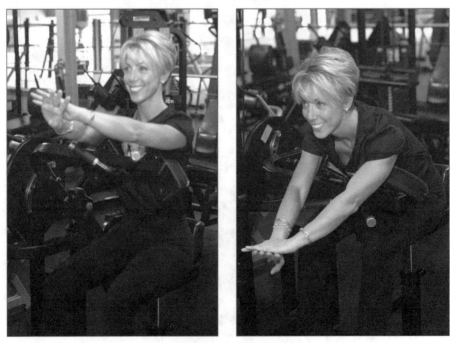

Abdominal machine: Abdominals

Advanced Routine II

This routine utilizes the half-rep principle. This advanced procedure uses a half rep followed by a full rep. Meaning that, from the starting position, you perform only half the motion. For example, with a bicep curl, a full rep requires you to bring the weight from your thighs all the way up to your shoulders before returning to the starting position. A half rep would require you to stop the lifting motion half that distance, when your forearms are perpendicular to your body, then return to the starting position.

This routine uses a half rep followed by a full rep as one complete repetition; the combination should be counted as one rep. All exercises are to be performed in this manner. Never stop while you're doing an exercise (unless you're experiencing unusual pain). See all the reps through to the end, and then, without resting, go immediately to the next exercise.

To start, perform this routine one time through. When you can successfully complete two times through, you're ready to proceed to Advanced Strength Routine I.

- First set: 15 reps (heaviest as possible for 15 reps)

- Second set: 8 reps (add resistance)

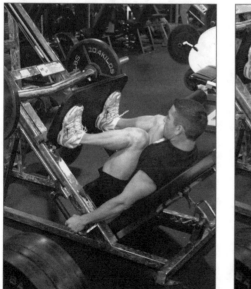 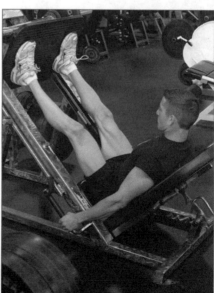

Leg press machine: Legs, hips, and butt

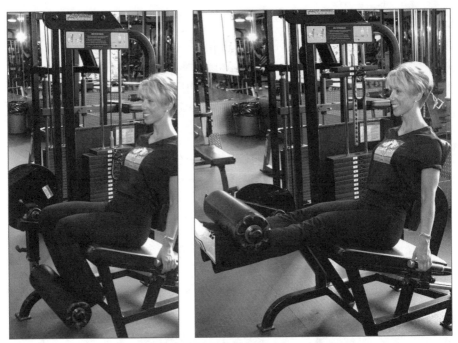

Leg extension machine: Legs, hips, and butt

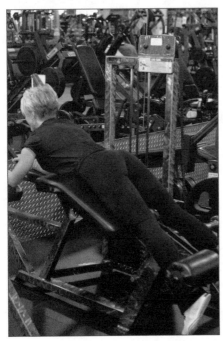
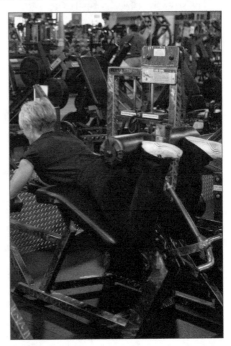

Leg curl machine: Legs, hips, and butt

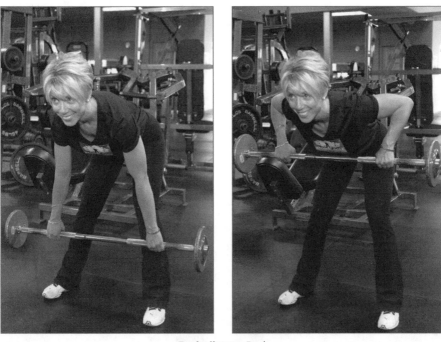

Barbell row: Back

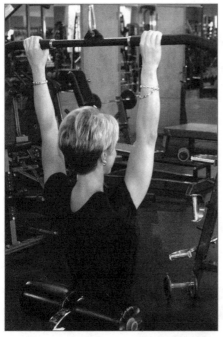
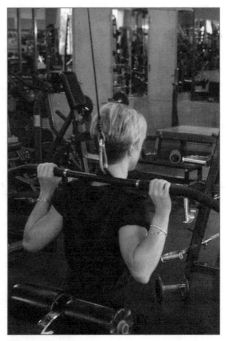

Lateral pull-down behind neck: Back

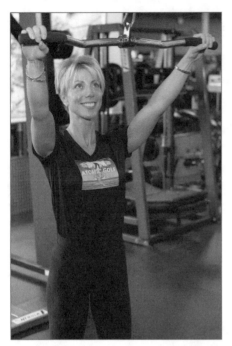
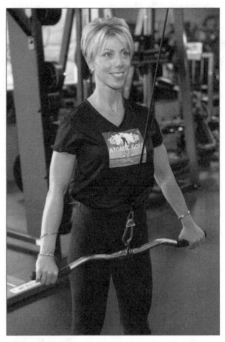

Straight-arm pulls: Back

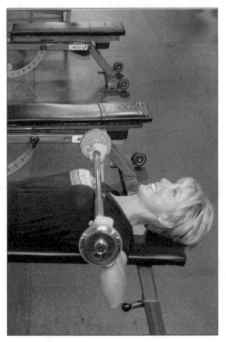
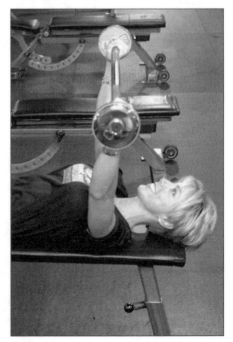

Bench press: Chest

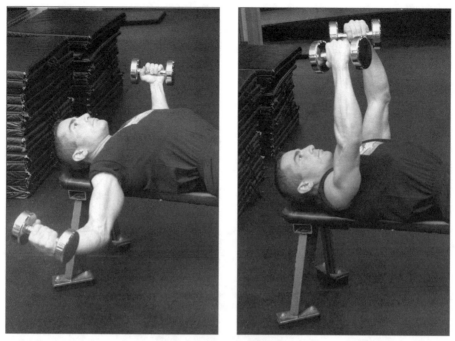

Dumbbell flies: Chest

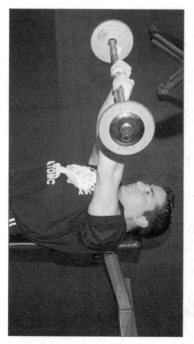
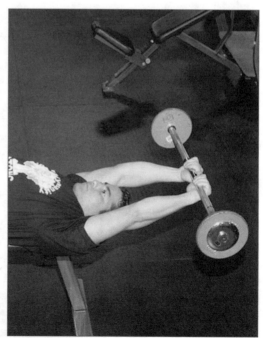

Barbell pullovers: Chest

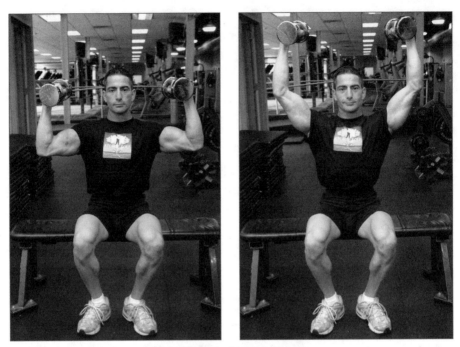

Dumbbell seated press: Shoulders

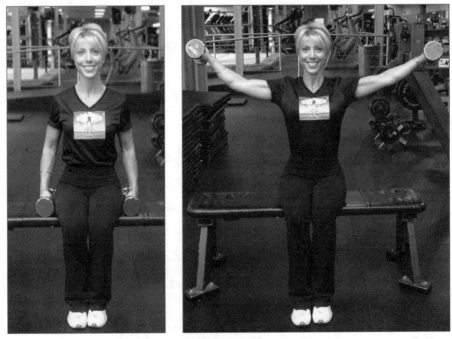

Side dumbbell lateral raise: Shoulders

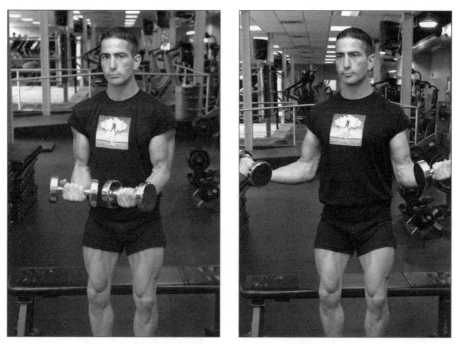

Dumbbell rotators: Shoulders

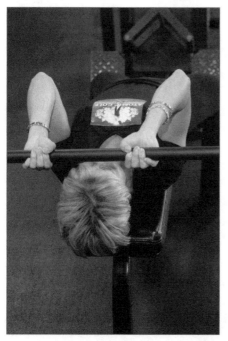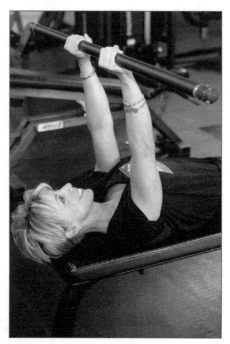

Overhead tricep extensions with barbell: Arms (triceps)

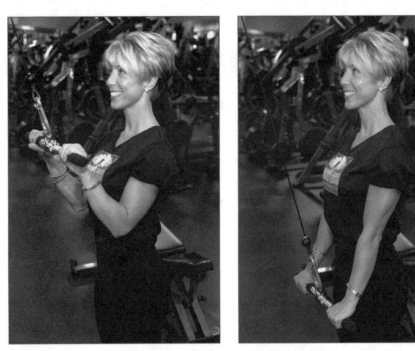

Tricep pushdowns: Arms (triceps)

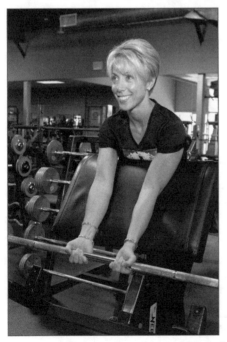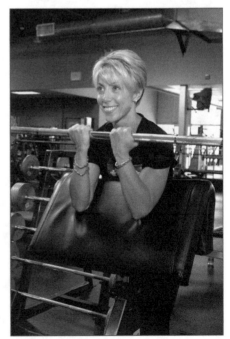

Barbell curl: Arms (biceps)

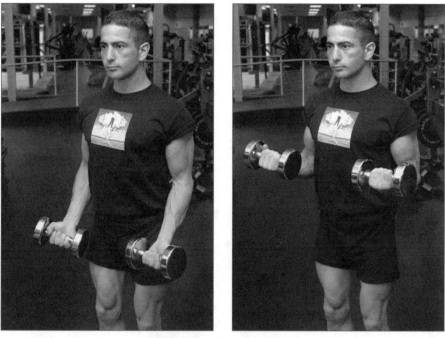

Dumbbell curl: Arms (biceps)

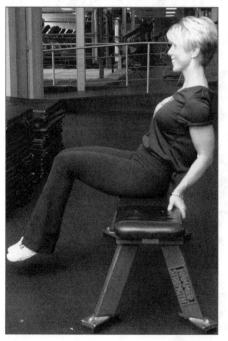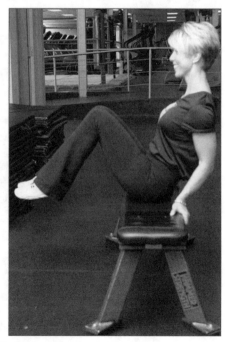

Knee ups: Abdominals

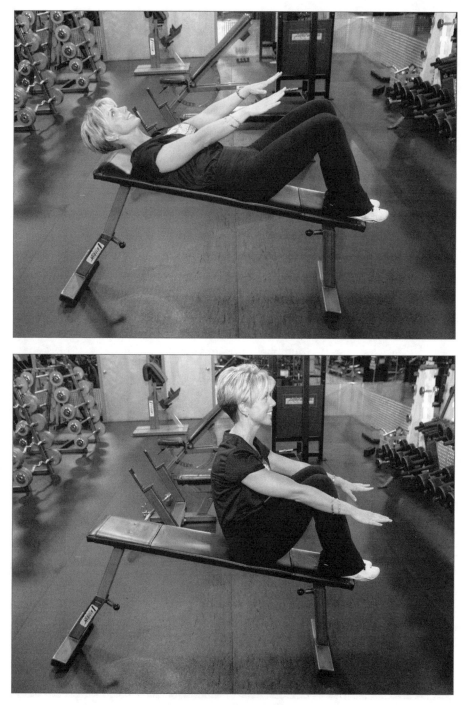

Bent leg sit-ups: Abdominals

Advanced Strength Routine

Perform one set of each exercise with eight repetitions. Do all the exercises one after the other, without resting, until the entire workout is complete.

- Start: Hold for 4 seconds
- Mid-goal: Hold for 8 seconds
- Final goal: Hold for 10 seconds

This is a static hold routine. It involves doing a complete repetition and then, on the way back to the starting position, stopping the motion halfway down and holding the resistance for four seconds. When you have mastered this, do the routine two times through for four seconds. Continue this pattern. Your final goal is to complete the routine three times through with ten-second holds. Once accomplished, you are ready to move on to Advanced Explosive Power Routine.

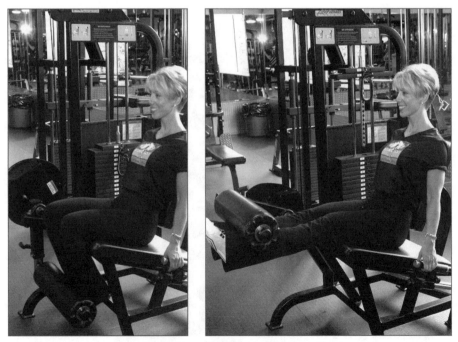

Leg extension machine: Legs, hips, and butt

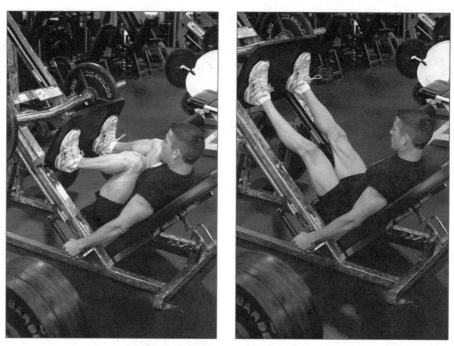

Leg press machine: Legs, hips, and butt

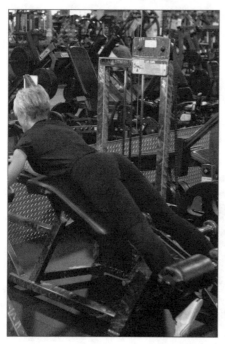
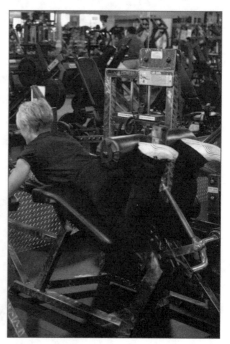

Leg curl machine: Legs, hips, and butt

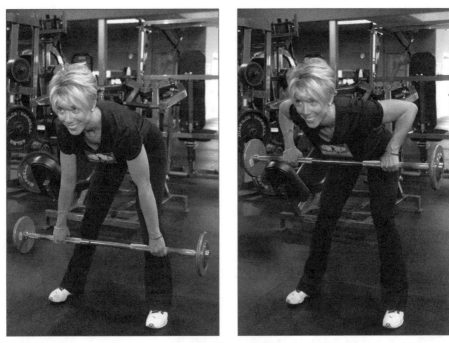

Barbell row: Back

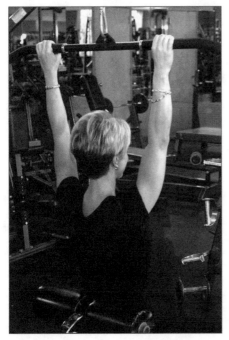 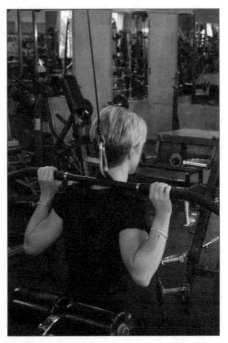

Lateral pull-down behind neck: Back

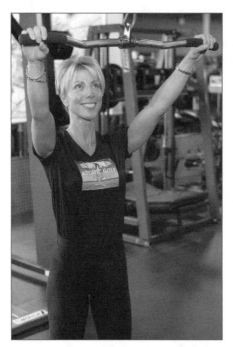
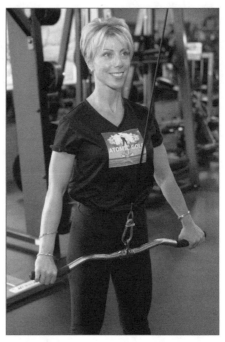

Straight-arm pulls: Back

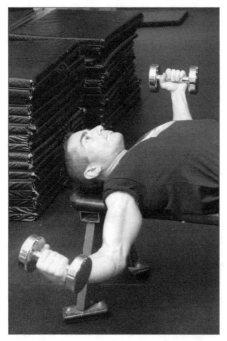
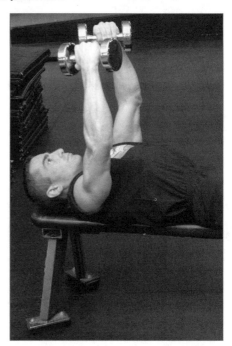

Dumbbell flys: Chest

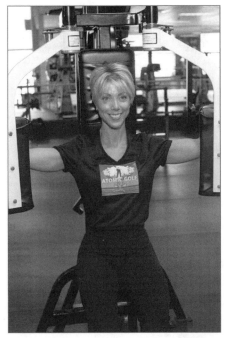
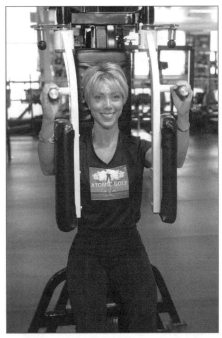

Peck deck: Chest

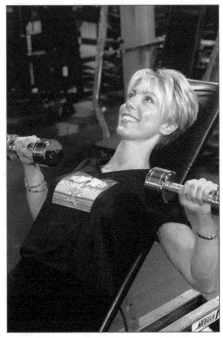
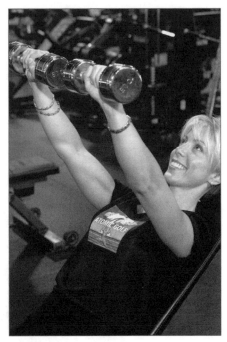

Incline dumbbell press: Chest

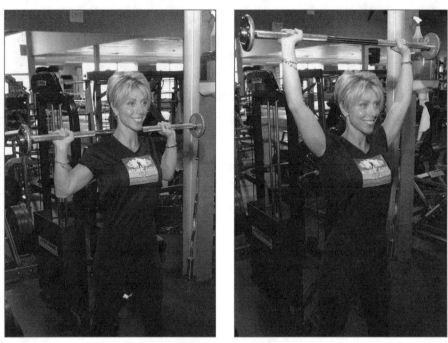

Barbell press behind neck: Shoulders

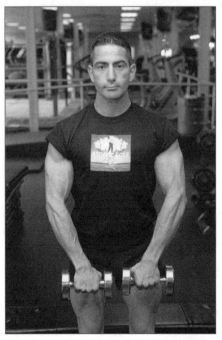 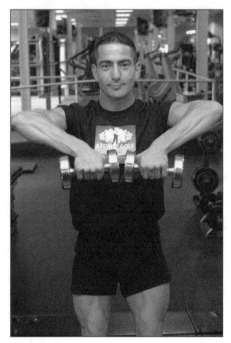

Upright row: Shoulders

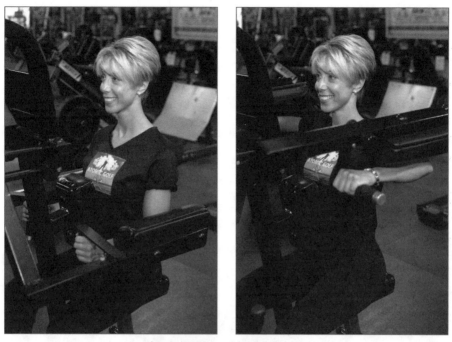

Side lateral machine: Shoulders

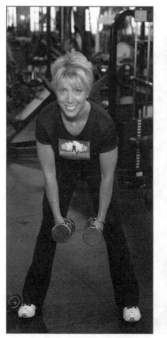
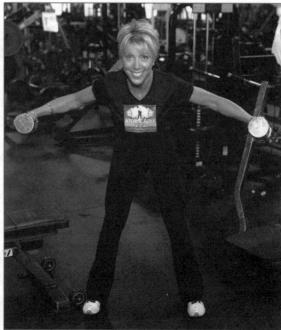

Bent-over dumbbell lateral raise: Shoulders

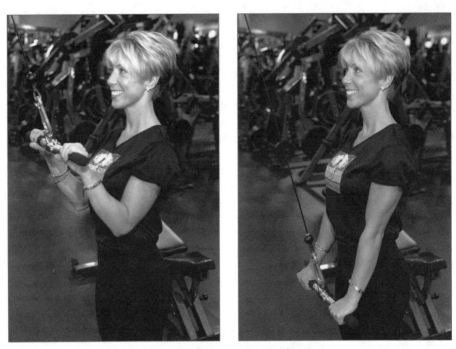

Tricep pushdowns: Arms (triceps)

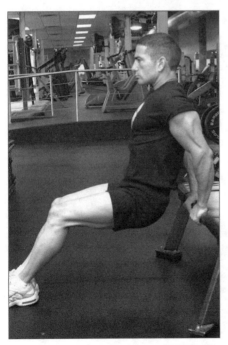
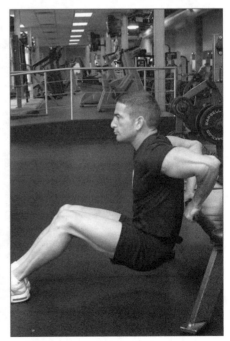

Bench dips: Arms (triceps)

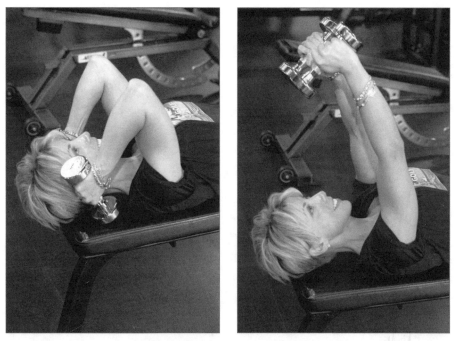

Lying tricep extensions: Arms (triceps)

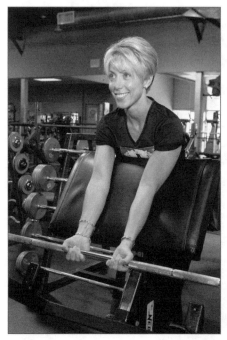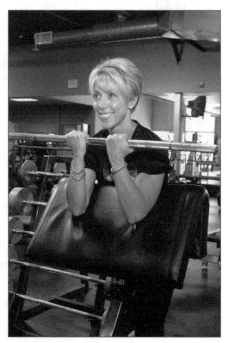

Barbell curl: Arms (biceps)

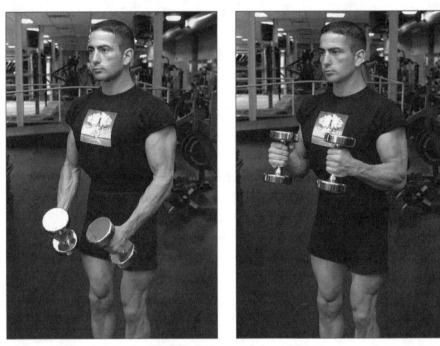

Dumbbell hammer curl: Arms (biceps)

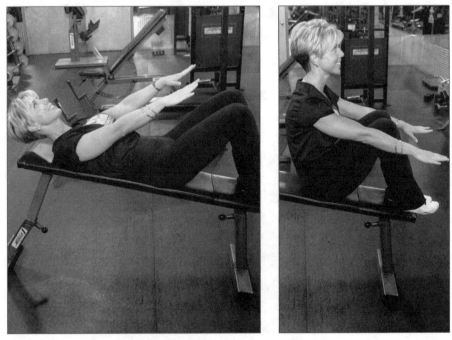

Bent leg decline sit-ups: Abdominals

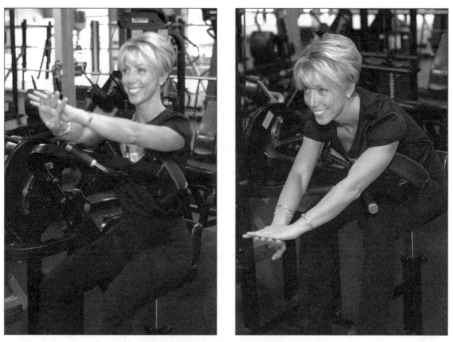

Crunch machine: Abdominals

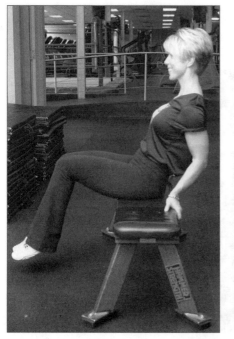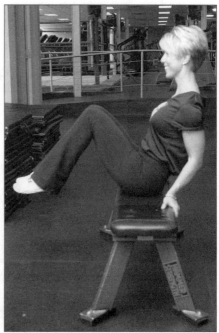

Knee-ups: Abdominals

Advanced Explosive Power Routine

This routine is called Stop and Go. It involves starting the motion of an exercise, stopping in the middle of that motion, and holding briefly before continuing to move the resistance the full range. This stopping motion is only performed on the initial range of motion. Do not stop the motion on the way back.

- Start: 3 sets of 10 repetitions (with a low resistance)
- Mid-goal: 3 sets of 8 repetitions (with a higher resistance)
- Final goal: 3 sets of 6 repetitions (with an even higher resistance)

Once you have mastered three sets of ten repetitions, continue this pattern. As the number of repetitions in the sets decrease, the resistance should increase. Your final goal is to complete three sets of six repetitions with the greatest possible resistance. When you are able to successfully complete this pattern, you are ready to continue on to Advanced Power Endurance Routine.

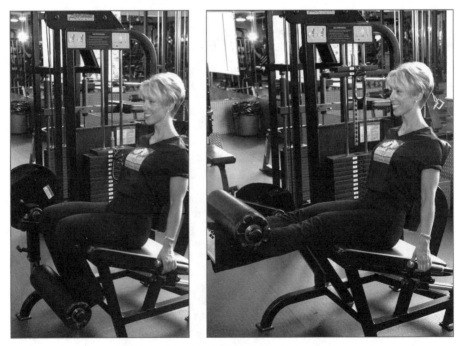

Leg extension machine: Legs, hips, and butt

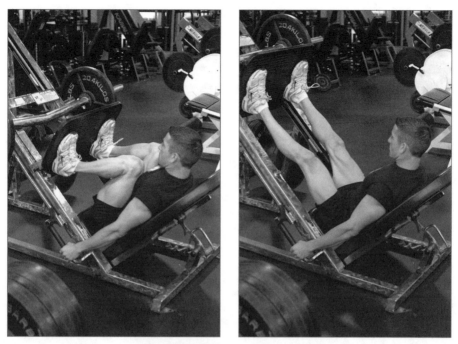

Leg press machine: Legs, hips, and butt

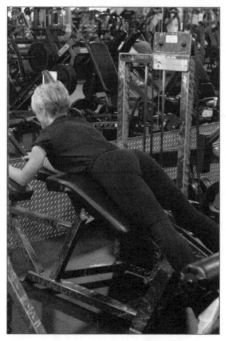 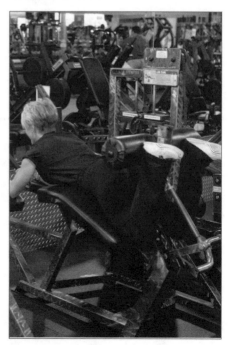

Leg curl machine: Legs, hips, and butt

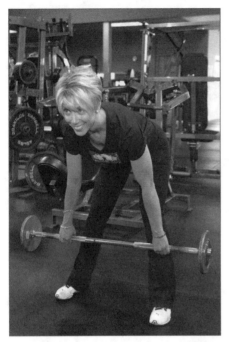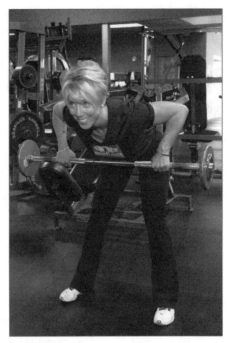

Barbell row: Back

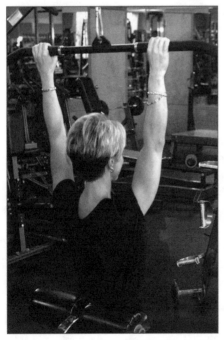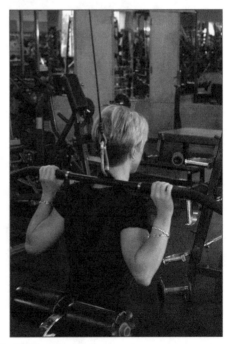

Lateral pull-down behind neck: Back

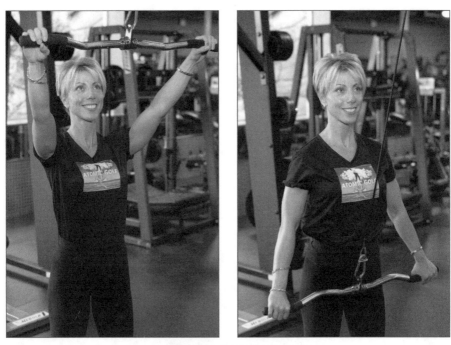

Straight-arm pulls: Back

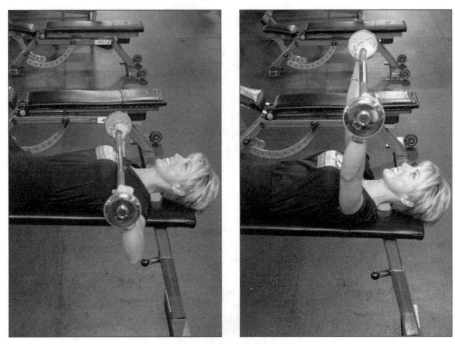

Bench press: Chest

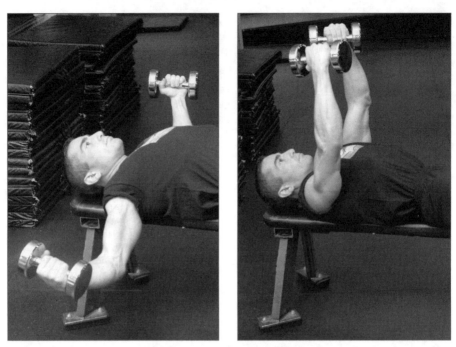

Flat bench dumbbell flies: Chest

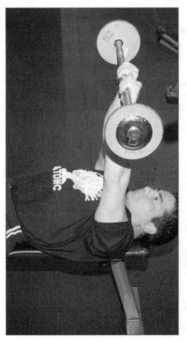
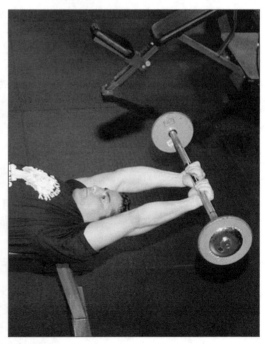

Barbell pullovers: Chest

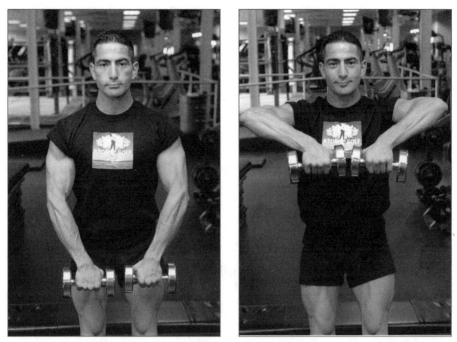

Upright row: Shoulders

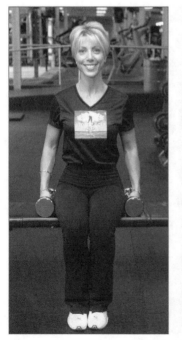
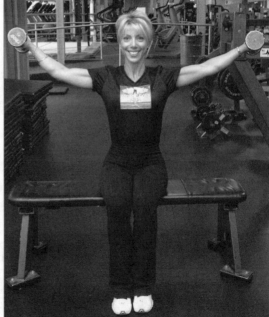

Side dumbbell lateral raise: Shoulders

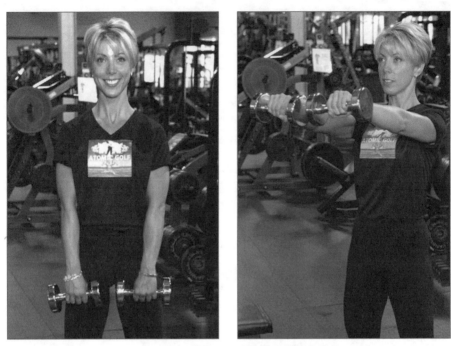

Dumbbell front raise: Shoulders

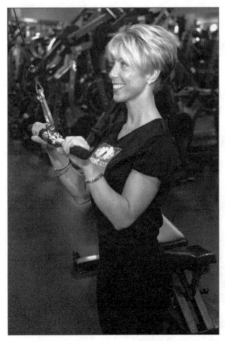

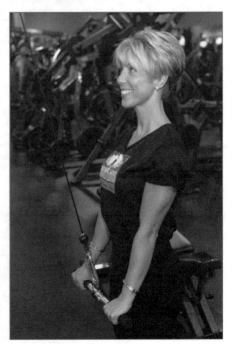

Tricep pushdowns: Arms (triceps)

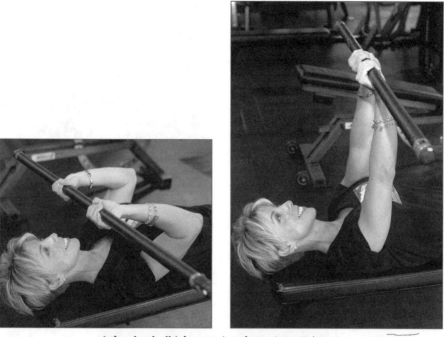

Lying barbell tricep extensions: Arms (triceps)

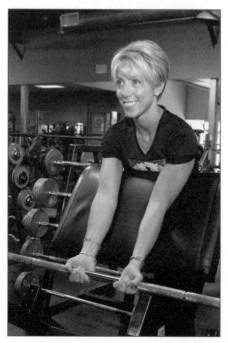
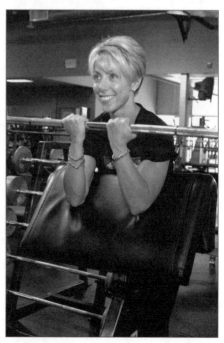

Barbell curl: Arms (biceps)

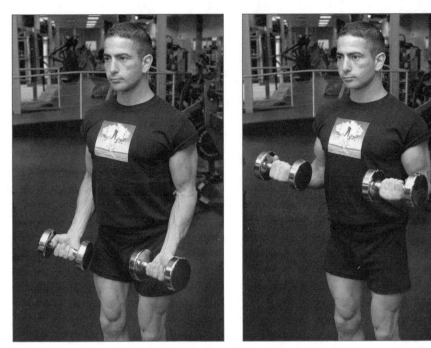

Dumbbell curl: Arms (biceps)

Advanced Power Endurance Routine

This routine has an aerobic component to it. Perform the required twenty-five reps as fast as possible for the first exercise, then go immediately to the stationary bike set at a high tension for three minutes. Continue this until all the exercises have been performed. Perform this cycle one time through only.

When you have mastered this, do a second cycle immediately. This time perform fifteen reps for each exercise.

When you have reached the ultimate level, you will perform a third cycle consisting of ten reps for each exercise.

- Start: 1 cycle of 25 reps
- Mid-goal: 1 cycle of 25 reps, plus 1 cycle of 15 reps
- Final goal: 1 cycle of 25 reps, 1 cycle of 15 reps, plus 1 cycle of 10 reps

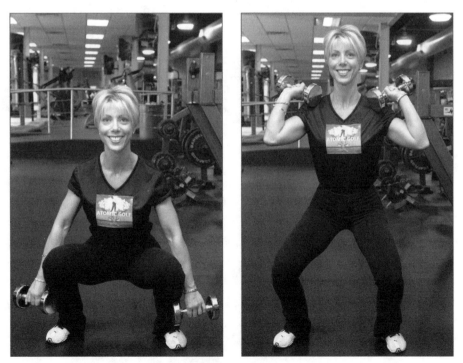

Power cleans: 25 reps

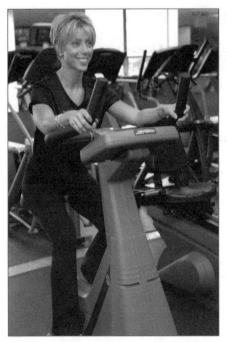

Stationary bike: 3 minutes hard

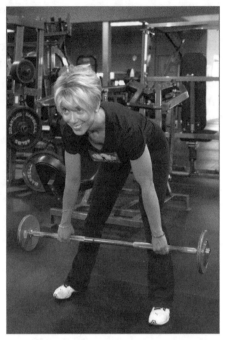

Barbell row: 25 reps

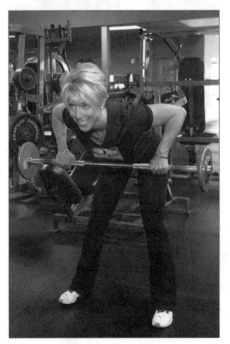

Barbell row: 25 reps

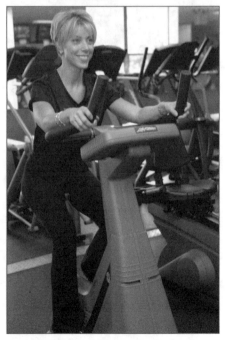

Stationary bike: 3 minutes hard

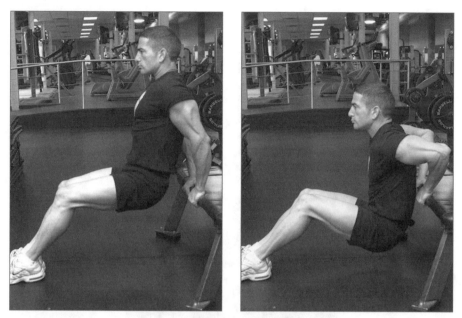

Bench dips: 25 reps

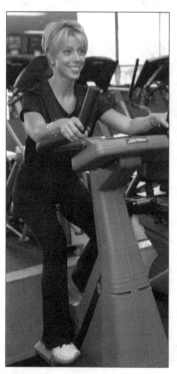

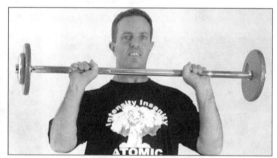

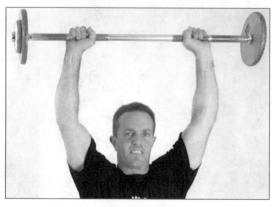

Stationary bike: 3 minutes hard   **Overhead barbell press:** 25 reps

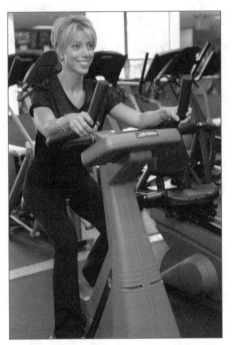

Stationary bike: 3 minutes hard

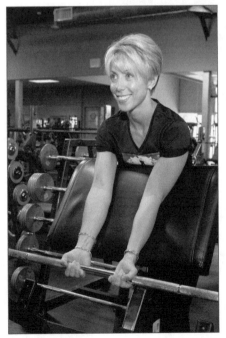 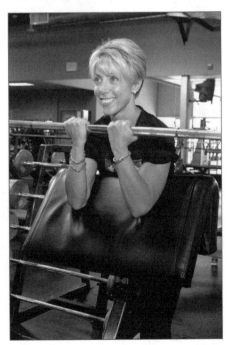

Barbell curl: 25 reps

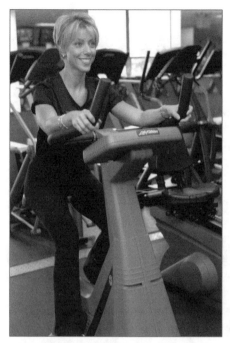

Stationary bike: 3 minutes hard

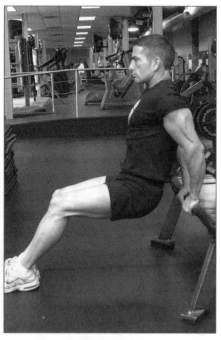

Bench dips: 25 reps

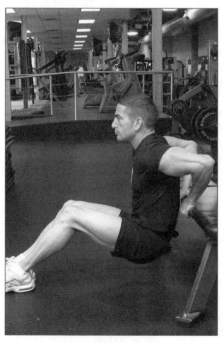

Bench dips: 25 reps

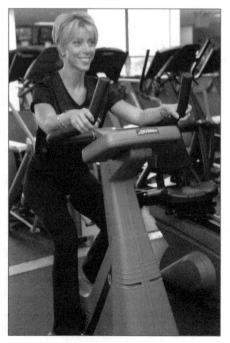

Stationary bike: 3 minutes hard

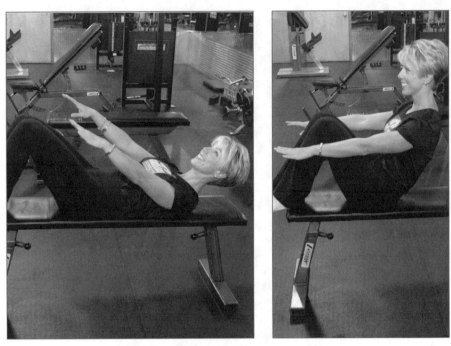

Sit-ups: 25 reps

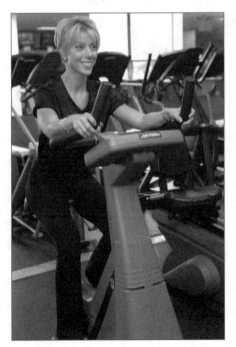

Stationary bike: 3 minutes hard

TROUBLESHOOTING

There are many reasons for failing or not achieving what you want in golf. We'll go through these reasons in no particular order. Each one is equal in magnitude to the other, and they all have a great deal to do with the sport.

1. **Fear of the future.** When you fear the future, you put yourself in a destructive game condition. When you are in this state, you infuse (to bring into) or are reluctant to reach out. When you fear the future, you do not maintain or enhance your abilities. You may stop yourself and others from doing what is positive. You will invest, on an unconscious level, your time, attention, effort, and resources into avoiding what you fear instead of what you want to achieve.

   Golf is played in the future. Many golfers treat the future as something they wish wouldn't happen. Their fear of not accomplishing their golf goals will inevitably produce a state in which they attempt to avoid seeing the future, for it becomes too agonizing to confront. Many losses or sad experiences of the past have to do with things that haven't really happened yet, but you believe will happen. Therefore, the attention placed on past loss creates inability in the future. A lot of athletes make present time the artificial end and miss the eternity of incidents ahead of them.

2. **Self-doubt.** Life is meant to be played in abundance. You have the right to be successful, and only you can make this happen. You are the creator of your universe, and every thought that you create will manifest whether you like it or not. You are the ruler of your destiny. You determine the mission and the purpose. You write on the great blackboard of life what is to happen. In golf, it is not the green, the club, the ball, the weather, or anything else that determines your success. You are the master of your universe. What you can envision and "hold in place" will happen in golf.

3. **Negative thoughts.** All events are manifestations of future postulates. Thought travels faster than light. All things are made out of light. All realities are a manifestation of light in some form or another. Thought is the reality of perception. What you perceive is what you believe, so what you put out there in front of you cannot go any other way but the way you wanted it to be. You program your future to be your present. You will pull in what you believe. It is the Law of Attraction. It is real, and you had better start to believe it.

4. **Lack of clarity.** Know your intention, and it will happen. Joy, peace, and success are only manifestations of your intention. You need to look at what you think and what you're projecting into your universe that is causing the failure. Find your position. The universe will open doors for you where before there were only barriers. Experience in your mind the feeling of winning, the exhilaration of success and joy. Put it out there, and it will become real. Let those old conditions and viewpoints go, for what you push against, you draw power to. What you resist will persist. In your golf game, you can't focus on what you need to overcome, for you will only attract more of the same. Instead, visualize only what you are going to achieve. See it. Know it. Focus on what you want, not what you don't want. The more attention you put on what you don't want in golf, the more of that you will attract.

MANIFEST YOUR DREAM

You need to know the fundamentals that changed me (Steve) from an ordinary person to a world-famous bodybuilding champion so you can do the same—and you can do this starting now. First, let me ask, have you ever asked yourself, "What am I? Who am I?"

As a human being, you are a composite of a being, a mind, a brain, and a body (BMBB). The degree to which these composite pieces are aligned equals an individual's ability or talent. When your BMBB is aligned, your talent flows uninterrupted. Of all the viewpoints I express in this book—without doubt—this one unlocks potential more than any other. It allows your skill, monetary income, and ability to soar. It took me a long time to comprehend the meaning of this, but once I did, there wasn't a contest I couldn't win. It simply is a matter of the being (you) perceiving the dream, seeing the vision in your mind, and commanding the brain (computer) to have your body carry it out.

You see, you must own the most basic fact known to humankind—that you are more than a body, more than a hunk of meat. You are truly an immortal being occupying a body. You may have dreams, but they may not necessarily be yours or your creation.

Once I realized that I had the ability to envision change, I could begin to visualize my own future. I had the power to perceive through imagination or thought. With this power, I was able to create my future reality. It couldn't go any other way. What I envisioned brought about my creations, not what or who I was. This, my friend, is fact—pure truth. You live in a universe that is connected to you. You are your thoughts. You cannot escape this fact. I am not a mind—I have a mind. The mind is a tool. I created that mind. I am not a body—I have a body to use. The body is simply a tool of the physical universe, different from a tree only in its purpose. I realized that I had a lot of say about the condition of my body. By bringing my dreams into harmony with my mind and my body, I was able to produce successful outcomes and win every major bodybuilding title to be won. This is fact.

By maintaining the alignment of my BMBB, I created this effect and overcame any and all barriers and problems. I created the belief system that would take me to the top of my game. I began to understand not only who I was, but also who I wasn't. Sure, I was born Steve Michalik, but that was a name and a title created by my parents and reinforced by others. For most of my young life, I bought into this identity. All my ideas for survival and solutions to problems were based upon being Steve Michalik—a fictitious character brought to life by others. Steve could never be fully in control. He manipulated life using preprogrammed ideas. I came to realize that the true being, the real creation and power source, was "me." "Me" has no name. "Me" occupies no space or time. "Me" has no form—it just is—and if truly awakened, it has the power to create miracles.

Once I really got this, my life underwent a paradigm shift. The energy surge was miraculous. I felt true power returning. I felt huge, and the veils of stupidity dropped from my consciousness. My life began to change incredibly. My body was able to soar to the purpose I put forth. My abilities increased enormously. My new paradigm became: I am—I dream—I visualize—I can—I did—I achieved all I wanted. The ramifications of this paradigm were vast. Not only did I realize who and what I was, but also I realized that this applied to all people. People clung to me, sought me out—it was magical.

You see, this matrix of factors comes into play knowingly or unknowingly whenever you undertake an action. To have ability, you must have the power to perform the action that produces desirable and useful results.

In essence, it comes down to having the ability to perceive what you need or want (the dream) and to bring the dream into reality. Once you have the dream, you must set up a model, a vision, of what is wanted. Then you must establish a plan to achieve your dream. Next comes implementing the plan that will make the dream a reality.

Let's not forget about quality of ability. After all, everyone has some ability. Examples of golfers who have obtained a high quality quota are Jack Nicklaus and Tiger Woods. When it comes to golf, they can accurately perceive what is needed on each of their shots. They intend to hit the ball to an exact place. They envision the model of where the ball will go. They plan how to hit the ball in the exact manner necessary to make it go where they envisioned it. And finally, they implement their plan to produce the desired results. Most important, they have been able to reproduce this consistently, game after game, year after year. This, my friend, is mastery.

You can apply this matrix to mastering any skill. If you can learn to perceive accurately, to form your intention, vision, and plan correctly, and to implement them accordingly to produce the desired results, you will demonstrate a high quality of ability in any discipline.

If you want to master golf, you must master the following basic factors:

- **Spirit:** You, the one who perceives what exists and what is needed and wanted.

- **Dream:** The intention, the goal, the target or mission—what you project into the future from present time.

- **Vision:** The manner in which you perceive something—the vision is the software of the mind.

- **Plan:** The detailed scheme, program, or method—the arrangement of details.

- **Implementation:** The act of fulfilling, performing, or carrying out the plan.

- **Result:** The outcome or consequence of the plan—the completed actuality of the dream.

- **Levels of existence:** The condition of your emotional and physical self—this will affect your present and future outcomes.

- **Belief system:** A set of related ideas, principles, rules, procedures, and laws of precepts that govern the acceptance or conviction of something perceived.

- **Life force:** The spiritual quality that propels particles and energy into space and time, along the parameters of one's life, thus bringing about the manifestations of the dream into the physical universe.

The quality and quantity of force alone determines the velocity of a dream's manifestation. This new belief system will empower you beyond your wildest imagination. Never forget:

The Dream

The Intention

The Vision

Plan It Firmly in Your Mind

Transfer It to the Brain

Implement It with the Body

Achieve Your Desired Results and Vision

THE TIME IS NOW

Looking into the future, *we* can see your final goals being realized. Now *you* must! Teaching old dogs new tricks may not be simple, but it is possible. Much bias and rumor plague our society. You must not be afraid to challenge current beliefs and see the light of the new, for all that is new is as old as the creation of the body itself. The principles we have brought forth are new only to the point of present understanding. The body and mind work a certain way—this is absolute truth. The mind follows exact rules of behavior regardless of your intentions. You must conquer with understanding what in the past seemed unconquerable. You must come to know reality and see it! Live it! You must have a love of life so profound that you become one with all. Be responsible to yourself. Seek truth and knowledge will follow. Then and only then will you finally be in control!

Limitations exist; this is true. Heredity cannot be changed. But if you understand the interrelationship of the body, the mind, and the method, then and only then can you make great strides in the direction of creating and demonstrating Atomic Golf. You must not repeat the errors of those who fail to recognize the benefits of exercise toward golf. There has existed an obvious blind spot, even in medicine, that's finally being lifted regarding the benefits of conditioning the body. For years, doctors (who incidentally, die younger than most other professionals), rejected what we have been preaching. Although these biases still exist, the facts are self-evident and should not be ignored. Nor is it necessary to obtain a degree in biophysics in order to make practical use of these facts. We have attempted, in as simple a manner as possible, to outline the basic points of knowledge and the principles of application necessary to produce the ultimate result: the Atomic Golfer.

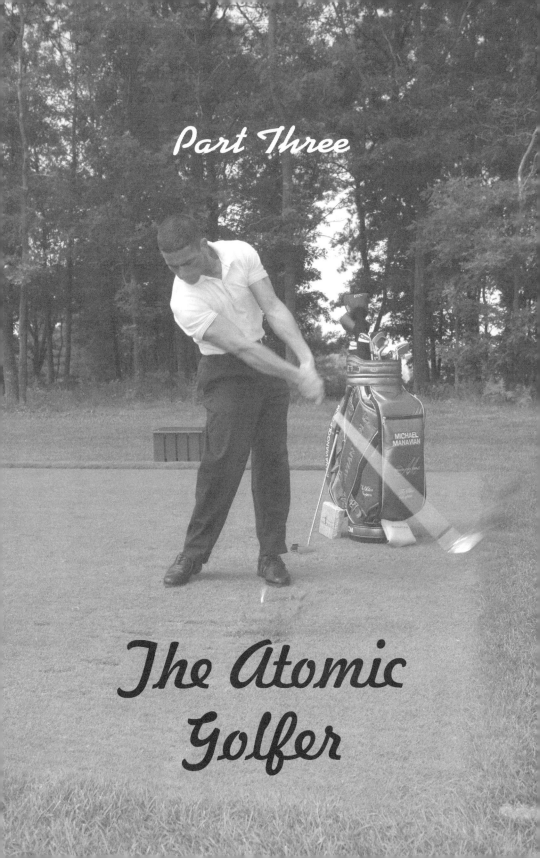

Part Three

The Atomic
Golfer

The Origins
of Atomic Golf

"**M**r. Manavian, where are you going to work when you graduate from here?" quipped Jerry Hogge, my professor at Methodist College.

"I am going to get the *perfect* job," I responded brashly.

Well, this really fired up my professor, who replied with a scoff, "Don't bother, they don't exist."

From that moment on, my total focus for the remainder of the semester was to make my goal a reality, despite my professor's viewpoint. I started to look at what could be the perfect job within the golf industry. What could I do that would create the biggest effect in other people's lives? I deduced there was no greater reward than to show someone how to successfully play this great game of golf.

After graduation, I was hired to fill a teaching vacancy at an extremely busy facility in Connecticut, within an hour's drive of New York City. Many of my clients were Wall Street commuters, who had very little time, demanded instant results, and had no tolerance for failure.

Fresh out of college and only twenty-two years old, I was immediately thrown into the teaching fire by my boss to see how I would handle the workload. Needless to say, after four consecutive weeks of sixty-plus hours, in addition to a waiting list for cancellations, I had eased my boss's concerns. The sheer volume of lessons was amazing, and they happened at a pace that would overwhelm other instructors. My students couldn't buy renewal lesson packages fast enough! After a full year, I had given more than twenty-eight hundred golf lessons!

What I was teaching brought results unlike those of other instructors.

My clients were in shock at how simple it was to grasp the powerful concepts I used and duplicate them on the course. Especially those students who had sought out advice from the world's "top instructors" that money could buy and still weren't breaking eighty on a consistent basis. My students were winning their club championships and member events. I had rank beginners qualify for the U.S. Amateurs in six months! Others were being selected to represent their states in the National Team championships. It was very common to hear back from my clients after they had just destroyed the field in their father/son events or when full-time homemakers broke ninety for the first time after being stuck shooting in the 130s! This thrilled me just as much as when I learned of a student winning on the PGA Tour!

Because my lessons worked, my students were playing better and having more fun. I was even credited for saving a few marriages, as the husbands weren't so dejected when they came home after a round of golf. For as long as I can remember, I was born with an ability to fix other people's golf swings. For whatever reason, when I gave a tip or advice, it would create a positive effect in other people's games. But deep down, I knew there was still something missing.

I had spent all these years researching and perfecting what to teach and how to teach it but I had neglected my own game. My comfy little gig had turned into a liability. I was quickly approaching my twenty-third birthday and making a good deal of money, and yet I hadn't gone out and demonstrated my own ability in tournaments. It was time for me to experience the same thrill of victory my students were having.

REALITY CHECK

Knowing full well that I couldn't juggle a teaching schedule and play golf at the same time, I got rid of my apartment and all of my possessions except for my clothes and golf clubs, packed up my car, and headed to Florida to seek my destiny . . . only to be slapped in the face with the biggest reality check I had ever had.

My golf swing was perfect; it had been refined and tweaked over the course of eight months. It was now pure, yet my golf game was a complete disaster. How could I have failed? There was one thing I had overlooked. The machine making my golf swing was not adequate for the task at hand.

At five feet, seven inches tall and 128 pounds soaking wet, I was playing in mini-tour events where I would consistently find myself having to hit five or six fairway woods into the par-fours in any given round. What made it worse was that I was watching guys hit eight irons and wedges into the same holes! It was obvious that my lack of strength, size, and stamina created too great a disadvantage to overcome players at this caliber.

So eight months and $90,000 of my own money later, I found myself back on the rock pile in Connecticut teaching golf again: distraught, shaken, and with no confidence.

Then, out of the blue, I got a phone call from a former golf coach who suggested I travel to Long Island and speak with Steve Michalik. I was told that Steve was *the* guy who could help me figure out the physical and mental part of my game. Knowing how badly I had played that year, I was open to all suggestions.

So later that week, I made the trek from Connecticut across the Throgs Neck Bridge to Long Island and rolled up on Steve's house, where he just happened to be outside in his garage. I walked up and introduced myself and absolutely got barked at. "Who the hell are you? What are you doing at my house?!" The fear of GOD himself ran through my veins. Frightened and scared, I didn't know what to do as this behemoth of a man was on guard and ready to attack. I froze there, stuttering like a deer in headlights. Not a moment too soon, my liaison came running out of the house after hearing all the commotion. He had left out the little detail of my arrival to Steve, informing him that we would be having a meeting to plan out my golfing future.

Within the first five minutes of talking, I knew that Steve was "the man." He was and is what a champion embodies. He is the winner of numerous bodybuilding titles—but not just any titles: Mr. USA, Mr. America, and Mr. Universe, along with twenty-two others. He was Arnold Schwarzenegger before Arnold was! But in golf, it's one thing to be a champion . . . but what about creating champions? He has built over five hundred bodybuilding champions—and not just local titles, we're talking national and international titles like Olympias, Mr. USAs, you name it! He has Olympic sprinters in his stable of clients who have broken their countries' national records and Major League Baseball MVPs (Most Valuable Players). Steve's credential list is deep. So I was curious, how did he do it? What were his secrets? And most importantly, how could this help me achieve my goals?

The next day, I got that answer. I was to meet Steve at the gym at

6:00 A.M. sharp. I was so eager to start the process of developing my physique that I didn't get a wink of sleep. I was there fifteen minutes early, ready to go. Steve greeted me and there was very little talking; he was all business. He smiled, looked at me, and asked, "Are you ready for this?" I told Steve, that whatever it took to be a champion, double it, 'cause that's what I want thrown at me, I'm ready to be a champion!

MY ATOMIC TRAINING BEGINS

In precisely seven minutes, and into my third exercise, my body showed how pathetically weak and out of shape it was. My liver shut down, I got really dizzy, my eyesight got spotty, my legs got wobbly like spaghetti, and I barely made it to the bathroom to throw up. I was experiencing a sugar drop! Yeah, I was ready! About fifteen minutes later, when I started getting my senses together, I asked Steve how I did. "You were pathetic; I have sixty-five-year-old women who can train harder than you! Are you the role model of what a professional golfer is made out of?" And thus the baseline was established regarding exactly how out of shape I really was.

How was I going to expect to win on the PGA Tour if I wasn't in the best possible shape? After all, to execute one's desired golf shot, one must have total control of one's body—especially under duress. Steve's philosophy of mind over body, in combination with his Atomic weight training and conditioning program, enable one to gain mastery over the body even while experiencing massive amounts of stress.

Over the next eight months, my body started to quickly change, my workouts with weights got more intense, and my mind was focused on each rep of every set to achieve the established goal. There was no deviation of my mind. Whatever was thrown at me, I confronted it head on and *never* backed off. I wasn't allowed to back off. After all, Mr. Universe was training me, and *he* has never failed, which meant that failure was not an option on *his* shift.

I could see how I was shifting my body into a mode of compliance that I only dreamed of. In essence, Steve put such a demand on my body to perform exactly the way we wanted it to in the gym that anything less was unacceptable. We were at cause over my body's performance, and we created the effect *we* wanted. We didn't just move weights and do reps, we pushed and pulled and shaped the muscle to get the body to look and perform the way we wanted to under unimaginable stress. When he trained me, it would be quite a scene. The entire gym would stop and stare in disbelief at the things I was able to do at Steve's command. One hundred-rep sets, two thousand-pound leg presses, and nonstop two-and-a-half hour training sessions were the norm. Now it was time to transfer this concept of mind over body compliance to the golf course.

THE MIND, THE BODY, THE SWING

At the end of this initial eight-month infusion of Atomic weight training, my weight had gone up from 128 pounds to 188 pounds of muscle. My body fat declined from 26 percent to 6 percent. My diet was functional versus sporadic, my high blood pressure and high cholesterol went down, and my golf game? Well, I improved across the board by 13 percent. Pre-Steve, my longest drive ever was 296 yards, now my long drive is 406 yards (June 13, 2008, Long Island Open, Bethpage Red, 18th Hole). I even entered a long-drive contest and finished fifteenth out of six hundred competitors. Now I consistently hit the ball in the 300- to 330-yard range versus 250 to 280 yards. I have limitless energy during my rounds, especially coming

down the stretch on holes fifteen to eighteen. I'm never tired. I can walk fifty-four holes in a day and laugh about it, then go to the gym and train like an animal. And yet my flexibility and golf swing have not been compromised, just enhanced.

I'm a bigger Mikey. I've got more mass, more functional muscle, and total control over my body 100 percent of the time.

Looking back, I was oblivious to the significant role my body and mind played in my golf game. Having gone through the mental and physical barriers myself, now I look back and see how twisted the world of golf has become. Steve and I have destroyed the myth that weight training is detrimental to one's golf swing. I am living

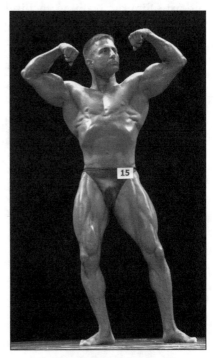

Golfers *can* build muscle.

proof that you don't need to hit thousands of golf balls a day to step on the first tee and shoot par or better. Learning to use the mind to demand compliance out of the body in a gym setting, where you are asking it to produce results while under tremendous amounts of stress, makes stepping onto the first tee and hitting a little white ball a cakewalk in comparison.

Up until now, the golf world had not made this mind/body connection. For the few golfers who have just recently caught the fitness craze, their exercise regimens are apt to consist mainly of stretching, which does little to improve their game and mental focus. These are the golfers who exercise—a meaningless activity that moves weights around and gets them tired and therefore they actually play worse! I have walked through the locker rooms of PGA Tour events; they are full of candy, sodas, and kegs of beer, with the occasional fruit platter laid out for display. Recently, Steve and I walked into the Tour's "fitness trailer" to check out what was available to these fine professionals. It was a shame to see what this trailer was composed of, given the abundance of discretionary dollars the Tour has at its disposal. Their fitness trailer made my weight bench, which is gathering dust in my attic, look like a forty-thousand-square-foot, state-of-the-art Olympic training facility! Steve and I couldn't stop laughing! It looked like a morgue on wheels! It's no wonder why the average Tour player looks like a penguin! From the top of the money list to the bottom, there is not one golfer on any tour who would meet the criteria set forth in this book as it relates to having functional muscle and an effective diet.

The Atomic Golf System is what creates real changes in the body and mind by taking it to the next level. Welcome to the world of "training"—a level where one demands compliance from the body.

13

The Atomic Golf Swing

*F*or as long as I (Michael) can remember, all I ever wanted to be was a champion golfer. As a young boy caddying at Oakley Country Club just outside of Boston, Massachusetts, I would envision myself holding that trophy on the eighteenth green and smiling for the photographs. I would pedal on my bicycle to all the local tournaments to get a glimpse of the top area pros, and when I got back home, I'd do my best to emulate their graceful and powerful swings. I can remember vividly waiting with anticipation for Saturday at 4 P.M. eastern standard time to arrive so I could record the golf coverage and play it back over and over to see if I could decipher the elusive matrix-like code within their golf swings, a code that had eluded golfers for centuries. I knew full well that because of my small stature I would have to be technically superior to others in order to outplay them. Thus, my search for the truth about golf swing mechanics began.

SOAKING UP THE DATA

As with any good research project, I began by collecting all the data I could accumulate. I read every book I could find in our local library. Then I'd go to the neighboring town's library. When I had exhausted those shelves, I would sneak into university libraries and see what books they had. Then I would go to bookstores and read up on the latest techniques from the current swing gurus and keep track with the latest newsstand magazines. I would research archived magazines from yesteryear, looking for the secret. Then, when I got to my freshman year at Methodist College, I hit the mega-jackpot of golf libraries! It seemed like each and every volume that had ever been written about golf had been donated to the college to form endless aisles and aisles of golf data. I checked out each and every book there over the course of my first two years, researching every author, player, and instructor I could find—new or classic, trend or fad, including David Leadbetter, Butch Harmon, Mike Hebron, Jim Suttie, Hank Haney, Peter Croker, Homer Kelley, Percy Boomer, Eddy Merrins, Jack Lumpkin, Tom Tomasello, David Lee, Bobby Jones, Ben Hogan, Jack Nicklaus, Jim McLean, Harvey Penick, Curtis Strange, Lee Trevino, Jack Grout, Jimmy Ballard, Jeff Bailey—the list goes on and on.

This was just the tip of the iceberg. I sought out instructors all over the country who were willing to spend the time with me for a golf lesson. I wanted to be a sponge and soak up all the data I could before I made a decision of where I wanted to hang my hat. Unfortunately, everything that I applied inevitably led to a dead end. There was some degree of workability to each person's instruction, but the more I examined each element, the more it crumbled under the scrutiny. I wasn't looking for a Band-Aid fix; I was on a mission to build the machine of machines, armed to the hilt with the ultimate golf swing, ready for battle on golf's biggest stage.

When the dust settled and I was able to look objectively at the data that is available to the golfing public, I came to the conclusion that the sport of golf is in total confusion. If it wasn't, there would be a single how-to manual on the golf swing, and everyone would read it, apply it, and play golf. But every instructor has some random particle of data that they try to make fit. When it doesn't work—because it is based on a flat-out lie—it creates a dangerous downward spiral that leads students into golf purgatory. It only takes one piece of false data to ruin the most perfectly laid-out intention.

DEVELOPING THE ATOMIC SWING

When my research concluded, the development of the Atomic Golf System began in earnest by looking at what worked best or most efficiently in three specific areas:

- How to start the swing.
- How to change direction of the swing.
- How to finish the swing.

Using the data I had collected from the tests and research to answer these questions, the rudiments of the Atomic Golf System began to reveal themselves—and with an exactness I had never seen before in golf.

I discovered that the delivery system is just as important as the data itself. Having the data, or knowledge, to create the most efficient swing possible does not, in and of itself, produce champions. You must also know how to package the data so the student can learn the swing. In Atomic Golf, the delivery system has been perfected so the student constantly progresses with maximum gains. No step is passed until the previous step is understood with total certainty and duplication.

The unique discoveries of the Atomic Golf System are twofold. What is presented here is: 1) a 100 percent workable set of never-before-released principles that allows a golfer to have complete command of how they start, change, and finish their golf swing; and 2) a delivery system that perfectly sequences this information with checkpoints and drills along the way to ensure success. The Atomic Golf System is designed for the sole purpose of duplicating these powerful Atomic concepts with every shot.

The Problem with Golf Instruction, Golf Equipment, and the Lies You've Believed

*A*s an instructor, I was now armed with this powerful knowledge, so I began to run some beta tests on my clients. The results were nothing but perfect. Every student improved. Tough students, eager students, young and old, male and female, it didn't matter, they all had more solid structure at impact than before.

But I found that a new problem arose. It wouldn't stick in the real world. In a controlled environment like a lesson tee, I was getting these players to hit the ball super, and they would go out and play somewhat better, hitting better shots, but their scores wouldn't change. They would still "rollercoaster" during their rounds. Their golf swings on video were far superior to what they looked like before, but this too produced limited results.

GOLF INSTRUCTION

Enter the Atomic Golf System, which states that once you've learned how to efficiently hit a ball, any problem that arises is *not* from your golf swing. How could it be? Did you forget how to do it all of a sudden? You cannot fix your golf *game* by fixing your golf *swing*. Yet this is what the world of golf does. And I can't blame them. They haven't been able to find a professional instructor who's worth a dime and who knows how to build an efficient golf swing in every student, 100 percent of the time. This isn't even to mention the hundreds of dollars that these so-called experts charge for a lesson! So unfortunately, the playing public has been stuck in an endless cycle of bad golf with no chance of ever changing.

As a result, the golf instructor, over the years, has found himself to be in a bit of a rut. They are in a situation where there is an abundance of new golfers every year who want to improve, and all they have to teach these students is the same cookie-cutter, robotic rhetoric. The instructor's lessons typically last thirty to sixty minutes, within which time they hope to give the client something quick in the first five minutes that sticks and then to practice it for the rest of the session by repeatedly beating balls. If the student doesn't get it, they are instructed to go to the driving range and figure it out on their own.

As the "authority on golf instruction," the PGA of America has failed miserably to take responsibility in the teaching arena. The PGA cannot create a valuable product with its instructional techniques, despite all the technology available to it. There is no cohesiveness from one instructor to the next, and the handicaps of golfers haven't gone down in the past thirty years. The PGA should seriously look into adopting what is in this book if it is truly, as the motto says, "dedicated to growing the game of golf."

There are two possible explanations for the PGA's lack of effectiveness in this arena: either 1) the PGA truly doesn't know what it is doing in golf instruction, or 2) it is intentionally suppressing the information needed to help golfers get better in order to keep profits afloat. Bad golfers buy more lessons and more equipment, believing the answer lies therein—that is, if they don't quit the game first.

Now with this book available to golfers, never again will the search for an efficient swing be blamed for bad golf.

There is also the other type of golfer: the players who are a tad more accomplished and have been known on occasion to hit a perfectly struck shot toward their intended target. The tournament professional is one of these people. You can't argue that these players don't know how to hit a golf ball. They have succeeded where other people failed and found a way to get their ball where they want often enough as to make a living at it. So why is it that they still hit bad shots? One would think that a player like Vijay Singh—who practices more hours in a day than any other player on tour—would and should *never* hit a bad shot. But he does, and he has done it at critical times. Interesting, too, is the "solution" he applies. He heads straight to the driving range and beats balls over and over again.

At this level, where the motorized golf swing mechanics are learned, *the problem is not the player's golf swing.* It is rooted in his or her mind or body. If the player is not focused mentally, they are not totally in present time, controlling the body, and the body cannot play good golf on automatic. You have to be fully there, controlling and commanding the body. And if your body is not fit enough or well-nourished enough, it will dramatize the effects of hunger or tiredness and pull you out of present time, resulting in bad golf shots. Yet every person to a fault blames their swing and looks for more instruction, more video lessons, newer golf clubs, new golf balls, new golf shoes, new this, new that, and more! I am surprised more people haven't ended up in the loony bin because of these unusual solutions to a simple problem.

The advanced golfer's problem can be simply fixed by looking at how well their mind and body allows them to repeat the golf swing they already know how to make.

GOLF EQUIPMENT

People always ask me, "Well, what about equipment? What do you think of this ball? Or that driver? Which irons are the best?" My simple answer has always been that the best equipment available is equipment that is fit for *you*. My clubs are fit for me and no one else. The golf swing is like a fingerprint, and no two people have the same identical motion. Logically, then, it would make sense that no two people should ever buy the same set of clubs off the rack. Do not believe the hype! The major golf manufacturers are publicly traded companies that have shareholders who need to earn profits year in and year out. They are in the business of making money by selling you on the idea that their products will improve your golf game. While your equipment is definitely an important part of your game, will new equipment for the sake of new equipment improve your game? No. In fact, equipment comprises only 17.5 percent of your entire game. And that is only if your equipment fits you 100 percent accurately.

Golf manufacturers have major public relation firms working for them to get their word out. Take a look at the TV announcers you have grown to love over the years. You've let them into your living room for a few hours on Sunday afternoon. And every single one of them—bar none—has an equipment contract to hock goods. Jim Nantz does voiceovers for Titleist. Johnny Miller has been Callaway's pitchman for years. Gary McCord is in TaylorMade's corner. David Feherty is promoting Cobra Golf. The manufactures are not stupid. They do a wonderful job of promotion. But at the end of the day, all of their efforts can potentially only contribute to a maximum of 17.5 percent of your game.

I say "potentially" because the equipment they sell is off the rack. Would you buy a pair of shoes that wasn't the right size? Or buy a designer suit that didn't fit? Yet every single day golfers walk into a shop, after being ooh-ed and ah-ed by the latest TV commercial, and ask for a certain name-brand product!

By the end of this section, you will be armed with the information and knowledge needed to find yourself a clubfitter near you who will be able to build a set of clubs that will match your swing using the best technology available.

DRIVING RANGES AND GRILL ROOMS

I would be amiss to not touch on those pessimists who linger on the driving ranges and in grill rooms all across the country; those golfers who cannot confront their inabilities and have given up hope of ever improving their games. They believe they will never get better and agree that golf is a "hard game" that can never be mastered. This book takes their beliefs and shoves them right back at them! Do not fall into the same trap they have, for you *can* improve your game. You have taken the first step and gotten this book, where all the tools of truth have been given their rightful sequence, ready for your mastery.

So read and apply everything in this book. You have our personal guarantee as authors that it will keep the men with the straightjackets at bay.

THE TRUTH ABOUT FALSE DATA

I've seen it all too often. Eager and willing students thumbing through the latest issue of a golf periodical with hopes that some "newfound secret" is going to revolutionize their golf game forever. They read the information, practice it, read it again, show it to friends, check with their pro, head to the driving range, and magically, poof! It works! To their amazement, it worked on the first try. They tee up another ball, swing away, and thwack! A slice followed by a hook, then a shank and top. That ingenious bit of data from the magazine didn't duplicate itself. The golfer starts to blame himself or herself. Thinking it was their fault (how could a magazine be wrong?!), they take these thoughts to the course and rollercoaster up and down from shot to shot, not knowing which way is up, only to find themselves dejected and hopeless. That is, until they realize they are only thirty days away from the next big magazine secret!

This is not a parody, but an actual cycle of action that is the norm in the minds of many golfers.

The truth is, about 99 percent of all the data available out there on the subject of golf is false and unworkable. And the other 1 percent, which is workable, usually isn't aligned properly to get the intended result.

The law of attraction is always working. This law states that you create what you put out there, meaning that your postulates determine your experience. If what you put out there is a vision of a golf swing that is loaded with false data, you will create a poor shot. Applying false data has a very definitive outcome. You are not going to suddenly produce an optimum shot. Conversely, just by understanding these true precepts about the golf swing, you will create the optimum golf shot.

Note that I used the word "optimum." By this I mean maximum energy transfer in the intended direction.

Tiger Woods plays at this level. His swing speed is 125 miles per hour (mph) with a ball speed of 190 mph. Do the math: $190/125 = 1.52$ efficiency rating and a ball hit more than 300 yards.

In contrast, John Q. Duffer will swing 100 mph and launch the ball at 125 mph, creating a 1.25 efficiency rating. And maybe he'll hit the ball just over 180 yards (a carry of 180 yards, that is, or how far the ball was hit in the air only, minus the roll.)

No matter how much you practice, false data will hold you back from playing your potential.

Your ability to attain clubhead speed and maximum energy transfer depends on your understanding of the direction of the clubhead toward its final destination.

For example: If you were to hammer a nail into a two-by-four, it would be in the best interest of your thumb if you proceeded to drive the head of the hammer straight into the nail head. Most golfers are trying to hit the wood! *Ouch!* Wrong target!

Hit the ball with your clubhead—don't try to swing it to the flag!

Another misconception is to swing the club and let the ball get in the way. If I was framing a house and I told my foreman that I was going to swing the hammer from 8 A.M. to 5 P.M. and hope that the nail got in the way, I think I would be fired by lunchtime.

This may sound funny, but it is an all-too-common belief in the world of golf.

There are tens of thousands of bits of information like these two examples, if not more, floating out there in the subject of golf. If you are stuck to any piece of false data and believe it is true, you are certain to find failure.

Look no further; this and only this is why you have not reached your potential in golf.

The lessons in the coming chapters are designed to help you look at the data you have accumulated and begin to remove the pieces that have held you back. Then and only then can you put in place the true workable data you need to succeed.

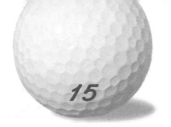

Atomic Golf Lessons, 1-6

*E*very discipline has its own distinct vocabulary. Golf is no different. Before we begin with the instruction phase of this section, it is important to define the words we are using in order to avoid any misunderstandings or confusions.

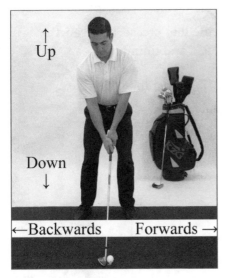

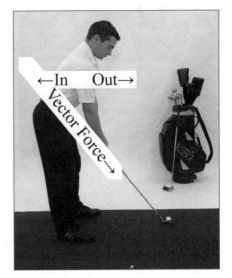

- forward: destination of the ball
- backward: opposite direction of the ball's destination
- up: toward the sky
- down: toward the earth

- in: direction from the ball to your body
- out: direction away from your body toward the ball
- vector force: direction of energy

- clubhead: striking portion of the golf club

- toe: portion of the clubhead furthest away from you

- heel: portion of the clubhead closest to you

- shaft: connecting tube between the clubhead and the grip

- grip: handle of the golf club

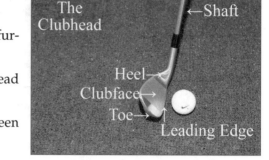

- leading edge: forward bottom part of the golf club that makes contact with the earth first

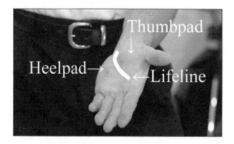

- heel pad: meaty portion of the outside of your hand

- thumb pad: meaty portion of your hand below your thumb

- lifeline: crease between the heel pad and thumb pad

- stance: starting position for your body in preparation to strike

- unloading: release of the golf shaft's energy

- loading: the action of storing energy into the golf shaft

- throwing: the action of releasing the golf shafts energy with the vector force

- balk: vector force with no release

- drop: release with no energy behind it

- inline: joining of two objects in a single axis line

- extension: straightening of the arms

- divot: chunk of turf torn out of the ground as a result of a properly executed shot

- spin: rotation of the golf ball around its axis

- impact: collision of the clubhead with the golf ball

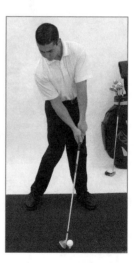

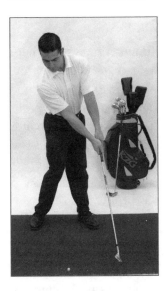

- follow-through: moments after impact when the arms are fully extended ◀

- backswing: backward movement of the golf club in order to store energy ▶

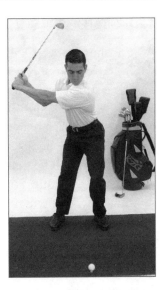

- downswing: (actual, at high speed) downward movement of the golf club, releasing energy ▼

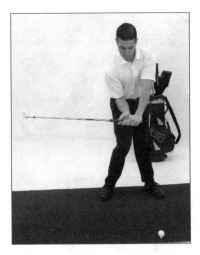

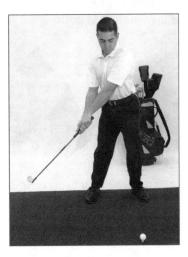

- downswing: (intention—at slow speed) downward movement of the golf club, releasing energy; what it looks like if you were to make a swing and view it in slow motion—without speed your intention would be only to do the slow speed one ▲

- agreed belief: a concept you have agreed to that unconsciously determines all associated actions.

THE STUDENT'S VIEWPOINT

As you start Lesson One, take the viewpoint of a student, one who is there willing to learn, not just there to accumulate more data. As each bit of information is given, carefully consider it and see how you can apply it. Also, as a student, understand that you do not know this data yet. This viewpoint will put you in a state where you are open to accept the information at hand.

Unlike other books on golf instruction, where you read pie-in-the-sky theories, you will be getting a golf lesson from the author—one on one! If you answer each question I ask truthfully, and do the drills that I ask you to do diligently, you will make the Atomic Golf gains as promised.

Strap in and let the journey begin!

REQUIRED TOOLS

To receive the maximum gains out of your Atomic Golf lessons, having the following list of equipment at hand is of great use:

- Golf balls
- Golf club
- Mirror

- Swivel chair
- Tees
- Tennis racquet

- Video camera
- Wiffle balls
- Wooden yardstick

In learning any activity, drills enable you to turn a conceptual understanding into knowledge. The demonstration of these drills shows competence and ability in what you have read. It is through the drills that learning the skill is accomplished. When doing these drills, put your attention on doing them exactly as intended instead of rushing through them for a quick result. Everyone's learning is based on understanding, not time. Once you get it, you get it, there's no benefit gained by overrunning a drill.

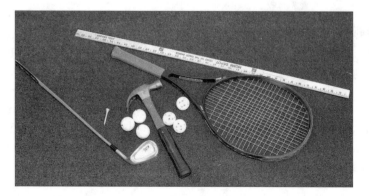

LESSON ONE: IMPACT

Read the question, and then write your answer in the space below.

Q. What would you like to get out of your first golf session?

A. _____

_____

_____

Q. If at the end of the first lesson, you were able to understand how to hit the ball up, straight, and forward, would that be a good start for you?

A. _____

_____

_____

Q. Let's have you hit a few shots and record them using the video camera, or chip a few balls in front of a mirror. As you watch the replay, use the space below to note what you like about your golf swing. Were you able to find anything you liked in your swing, or did you just make note of what you *didn't* like?

A. _____

_____

_____

Q. Let's look back at the video and take a look only at impact. When the clubface starts to make contact with the ball, what does your left arm look like?

A. _____

_____

_____

Q. If you were to draw a straight line from your left shoulder socket to the ball, does it trace directly over the entire left arm?

A. _____

_____

_____

Q. Is your left arm bent at the elbow? The wrist? Or both?

A. _____

_____

_____

Q. As you play the clip forward, frame by frame, does your left arm
   maintain extension through the shot, or does it collapse by continually
   bending more at the elbow or wrist joints?

A. _____

_____

_____

The purpose of these questions is to establish a baseline video. Whether you're a beginner who has never swung a club or an experienced tour pro, we now have proof of where you were when you started: good, bad, or indifferent. At this moment, we are not evaluating, rather we are accumulating data. We will come back to this marker throughout the book as the baseline swing.

There's a saying that if you know where Main Street is, you'll find a way to get there. At first it may not be the most efficient route, but over time and with repetition, you will be able to carve a straight path there. The same is true with your golf swing. If you know where impact is, then we can map the best way to get there. But if we bypass impact, you'll never get to Main Street.

A quick note on doing drills slowly. The slower you do a drill, the more precision you will need. How precise a drill needs to be is equal to how good you want to be. It is analogous to drawing a straight line; if you were to take a pencil and draw a straight line, you could do it quickly and draw it pretty straight because of the pencil's momentum. If you did it in ultra-slow motion, without the momentum, your hand might shake a little and not draw as straight a line. Point being, you need more precision when things are done slowly—this is where you will gain the understanding of each drill and teach your body how to do the drills. So take your time and really grind away at a super-slow speed. This way, when the time comes to add speed, your precision at these slow speeds will pay off tenfold.

As your instructor, I would not recommend you go to a driving range to "beat balls" at this juncture. Do all of these drills near a chipping green or in your yard, and really groove in these concepts.

Impact Drill I

Let's take a closer look at impact. Hold
your golf club waist high against a solid
object such as a person, pole, or tree, as
indicated in the photo, and move the
club forward as hard as you can. You'll
notice there is plenty of effort, but not
much power with that direction.

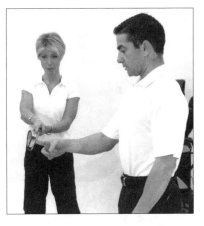

Impact Drill II

In our second drill, position yourself in front of the person or object, and
extend both arms and the shaft away from you into it. You will see that it
doesn't take much effort to force yourself backwards. Whether you're a
360-pound power lifter or a petite ninety-five-pound female, this direction
provides you with effortless power. You will transfer more energy away
from you than you ever will by going forward.

Now, looking back at your video, you'll be able to compare which of
these directions you are moving the club at impact. Are you maximizing
your power transfer into the ball by having this structured alignment of the
extended left arm at impact? Or is all of your effort being displaced? The
following drill will give you this desired structured impact.

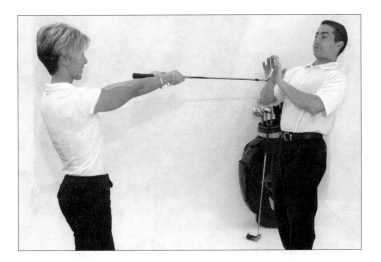

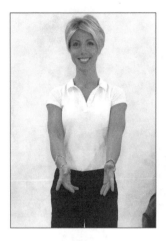

Impact Drill III

Without a golf club, stand nice and tall with your hands in front of you. ◄

Now take your hands and bring them toward your chest. Notice how your wrists and elbows collapse when you move your hands up. ▶

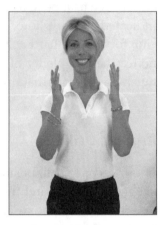

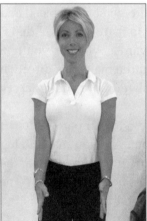

From there, extend your hands down toward the ground. Make note how by moving your hands toward the earth (down) that your arms are extended. ◄

Because of the biomechanics of the human body, your arms will extend when they travel away from you. You want this away direction to be toward the ball. ▼

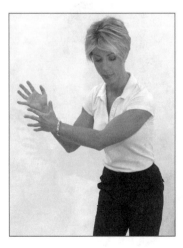

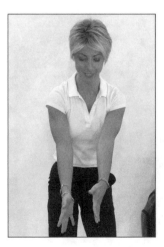

Extention creates maximum power.

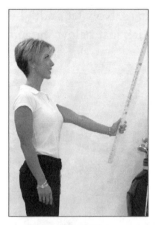

Impact Drill IV

Now take the yardstick and put it in your left hand. Hold the yardstick with six inches protruding under the arm as shown. ◀

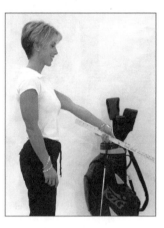

As if you were hammering a nail, move the tip of the yardstick toward the ground. ▶

Notice how, as you extend your arm, the butt end of the yardstick aligns with the underside of your forearm. Repeat this action five times. ◀

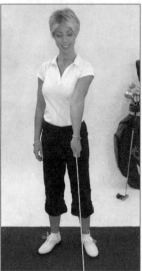

Now instead of hammering the yardstick straight down, move it back fifteen inches or so, and stop twelve inches past where the ball would be—at this point the yardstick should be inline with the underside of your left forearm. ▶

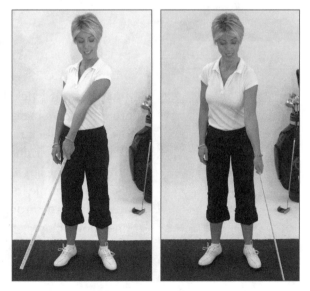

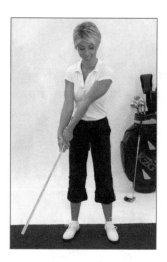

Repeat this action five times. Now let's add the right hand to the yardstick just below the left hand. ◀

Again, move the yardstick back fifteen inches and through twelve inches. ▶

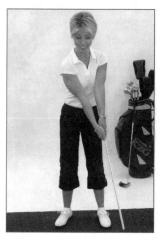

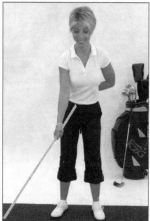

Did the yardstick align with your left arm, or did the right hand want to line it up with the right forearm? Repeat this action five times.

Now that we have educated the left hand, let's now educate the right. With your left hand behind your back, hold the yardstick in your right hand with eight inches protruding. ◀

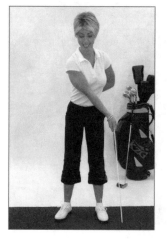

Move the yardstick back fifteen inches and through twelve inches. Pay special attention to how the yardstick must stay OUT OF ALIGN-MENT with the right arm, thereby being inline with where the left arm will be. You will notice this is very simple to do when downward pressure is applied through the proximal phalanx bone (bone closest to the palm) of the index finger—not the fingertip! Repeat this action five times. ◀

With both hands on the yardstick, feel how each hand now has to move through the impact area. Pay special attention to the right index finger's phalanx bone. ▸

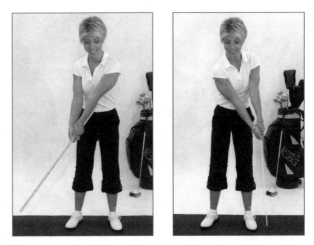

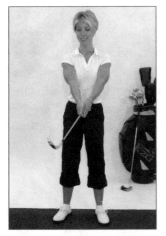

Each hand has a specific purpose; when done properly, you will maximize your energy transfer down the shaft and into the ball. You may even notice the better you move the yardstick into line, the more the yardstick will vibrate. Repeat this action five times.

Before you pick up the golf club, be aware of the extra weight of the golf club compared to the yardstick. Grip the golf club at the midway point. ◂

I want you to repeat the above drills using the golf club. Do these drills at about waist height. Be aware that if the shaft moves out of line with the left arm, you will catch yourself in the side of the rib cage—all the more reason to stay inline! Again, repeat five times each. ▸

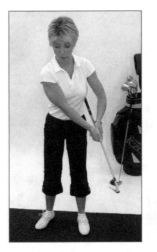
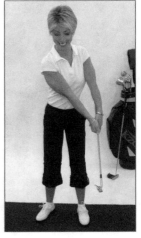

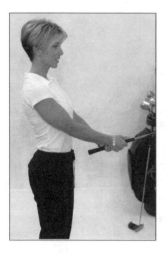

Now grip the club with 2–3 inches protruding. ◄

You are going to repeat the drills as earlier, except I want you to place a tee on the ground and hit the tee each time. ►

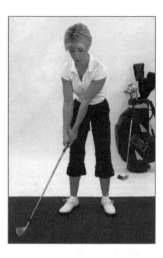

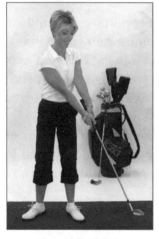

If you fail to hit the tee five times in a row, start over until you do. Demand compliance from your body! Once you have established certainty on impact with the tee, it is time to chip golf balls a short distance—no more than ten feet. Take your golf club and bring it back no more than eighteen inches and twelve inches through. ◄

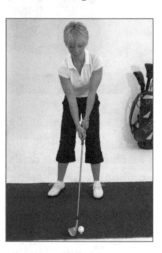

After each hit, check your structure. ►

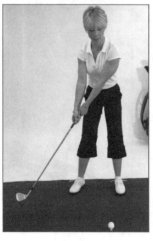

Is the shaft in line with the left arm? If yes, continue, if not, fix it and start over. Repeat this ten times through with certainty. ◄

This ends the drills for Lesson One. To gain the most out of this lesson, do the drills one time through the first day. Come back tomorrow and repeat the drills, this time twice through. Take the third day off, and on the fourth day do the drills three times through, bumping up the repetitions from five to seven, and ten to twenty, respectively.

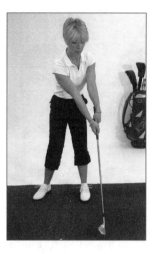

TROUBLESHOOTING LESSON ONE

If you notice, after doing Drill IV with the yardstick, that you're still having difficulty getting the shaft inline with the golf club, it's time we strip you of the incorrect beliefs you have agreed to accept. It is these incorrect beliefs that have stuck you in your bad swing for years. Your body will not process any new information until you break free from these agreed beliefs.

Q: If I were to ask you to hit a tennis ball up into the air, would the tennis racquet travel from:

a) Low to high   b) High to low   c) Level

A. *The correct answer is **a**. Moving the racquet from low to high will make the ball go up high into the air.*

Q. Now let's take a baseball bat and hit pop-ups to the outfielders. Would your bat travel from:

a) Low to high   b) High to low   c) Level

A. *Sure enough, again, the object would travel from low to high.*

Q. Now back to golf. To get the ball into the air, does the club travel from:

a) Low to high   b) High to low   c) Level

A. *The correct answer is **b**, from high to low. Because the clubface has loft, if you attempt to make the club go from low to high, you will put topspin on the ball.*

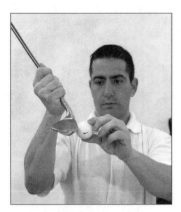

Look no further, this is the ONLY cause of topped shots, fat shots, whiffs/misses, skulls, and all other poor shots. If you were to correctly execute a swing that went from low to high, *you should miss the ball!* Unlike every other stick-and-ball sport, don't *ever* attempt to hit the ball into the air. Your only intention should be to take the club and hit the ball down into the ground just ahead of the ball. ◀

This will put backspin onto the ball and create the lift necessary to get the ball up. The more you attempt to hit the ball into the earth, the more the ball will go into the air. This is true with every club in the bag. In golf, down makes up! ▶

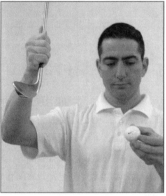

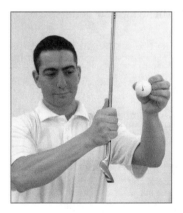

Let's go back to the drills. Before proceeding to Lesson Two, go back and repeat Drill IV with the new viewpoint that you are not trying to get the ball into the air. Rather, your intention is to drive the ball into the turf. ◀

By removing this agreed-upon belief you were stuck with, you will see a structured result in the way your arms travel through the impact area. ▶

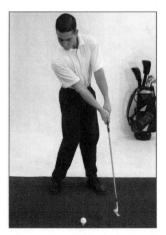

LESSON TWO: FOLLOW-THROUGH

Now that you have mastered impact to certainty, it is time to give you the next piece of the puzzle. Follow-through is the part of the swing after impact. From the end of impact twelve inches past the ball, ▸

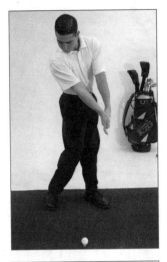

the swing continues to extend the arms down toward the ball, the momentum of the body forcing the hips to turn and face forward. ◂

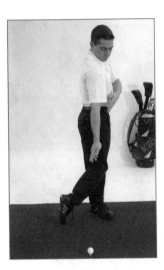

The final product of follow-through is a level body fully released from the impact position, with both arms extended straight down. ▸

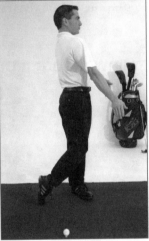

Follow-through Drill I

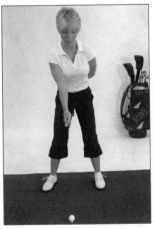

With your left hand behind your back, take your right hand to impact as you were during the impact drills. ◂

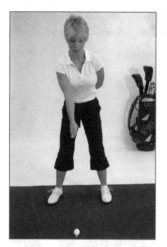

Add a little more speed, and see how by moving your right hand to the ball creates the momentum necessary to turn your body through the shot. (Note: Not *past* the ball, but *to* the ball) ◄

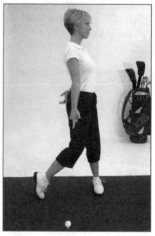

The better the right arm extension, the better your hips will respond by turning, and the more level your shoulders will be at the end of the drill. Your spine should be straight, as should your head and neck. You will be standing tall and proud with your right hand at the ball. Repeat this action five times. ▶

Follow-through Drill II

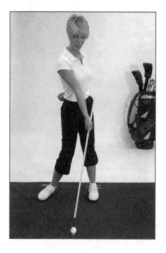

Now pick up the yardstick in your right hand, place your left hand behind your back, and repeat the exercise with the yardstick. ◄

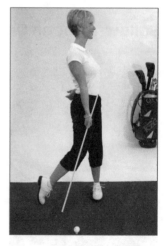

Pay close attention to how the correct motion of the right hand will move the body through the impact area. Just like in your right-handed impact drill from before, it is important that you keep the yardstick out of line with the right arm. ▶

Repeat this action five times.

Follow-through Drill III

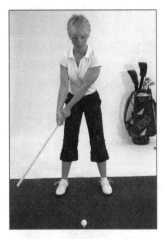

Grip the yardstick in both hands. Take the yardstick back no more than twenty-four inches, ◀

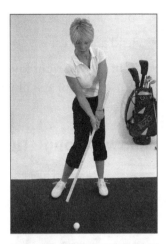

and down to impact, ▶

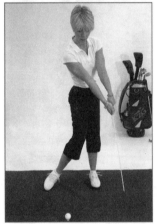

and from there slowly continue on into the end of the follow-through. ◀

You'll notice the difference between the previous two drills. Because your left hand is now also on the yardstick, you cannot leave the tip of the yardstick at the ball. Rather, the body movement brings the yardstick, and hands and arms, together in front of you as you face forward. Repeat this drill five times. ▲

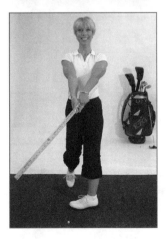

This is a critical step in the drilling process. Your reference points to check at the end of the drill are: ◀

• Shoulders: are they level?

• Arms: are they extended and below the belt?

- Yardstick: is it inline with the underside of the left forearm?

- Spine: is it vertical?

- Head and eyes: is your head facing forward with your eyes level?

- Right leg: the right knee should be touching the left knee, with the sole of your right foot at a ninety-degree angle to the ground, facing backwards.

Follow-through Drill IV

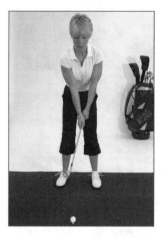

Moving along, take the golf club and grip it at the midway point of the shaft, well below the grip on the exposed steel or graphite. ◄

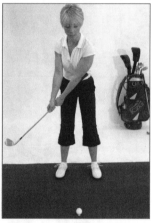

Repeat the exercise in Drill III above, again moving very slowly. ▶

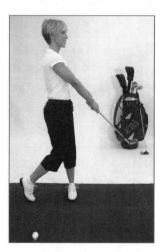

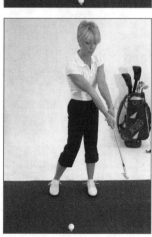

Note that with the extra weight and exposed butt end of the shaft, as you go through impact into follow-through, if you are out of line, the shaft will hit you in your ribcage.

Be sure to keep the shaft inline by extending down and to the ball. Repeat this drill five times.

◄

Follow-through Drill V

Grip the club this time on the rubber part of the grip with a few inches exposed on the back end. Stick a tee into the ground, and repeat actions in Drill IV above, this time hitting the tee. ▸

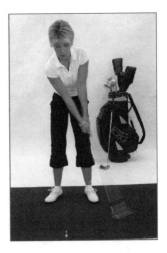

Repeat this drill five times, hitting the tee each time, if you miss the tee, stop and start over.

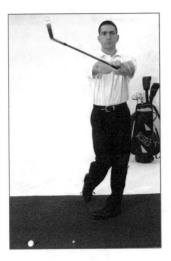

You will notice that an interesting thing happens when you add a heavier golf club later in the drills. With the added weight, you create momentum. This will force the arms to rise. ◂

This is a similar to what happens to a figure skater spinning on ice. The faster she or he turns, the more the arms want to flail out, though the more the arms flail out, the slower the skater will turn. In golf, in order to generate as much speed as you want, you must never agree with this vertical force, but instead fight it to constantly keep your hands close to the body, low, and below the belt. ▸

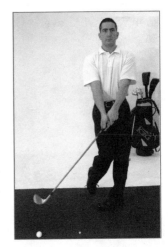

Follow-through Drill VI

Now it's time to chip some balls ten to fifteen feet off of a tee using what you learned in Drill V. Maximum gains will be made here by doing the drill slowly and completely. Grip the club at its full length and take the club back only a short distance—twenty-four inches max. From there, drive the clubhead from high to low, keeping the clubhead low and allowing the body to rotate into the proper follow-through alignment. Pay special attention to keeping the right index finger's proximal phalanx bone pressure downwards against the shaft.

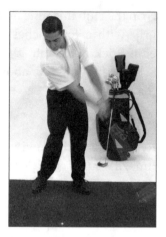

Repeat this drill ten times, hitting the ball each time; if you don't hit the ball crisply, stop and start over.

This ends the drills for Lesson Two. To gain the most out of this lesson, do the drills one time through the first day. Come back tomorrow and repeat the drills, this time twice through. Take the third day off, and on the fourth day, do the drills three times through, bumping the repetitions up from five to seven and ten to twenty, respectively.

Remember when doing these drills that speed kills! Make sure you go slow enough to get the correct alignments. If you add too much speed too soon, you will never, ever get the appropriate structure built in.

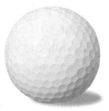

LESSON THREE: THE TAKEBACK

It's time to review the baseline video of your swing and see how you started your swing. Start at the beginning, before you have made any motion, and move the film frame by frame until you see something move then stop the video.

Put the numbers in their sequence as they moved in your swing.

1st   ___ Clubhead

2nd   ___ Shaft

3rd   ___ Hands

4th   ___ Arms

5th   ___ Shoulders

6th   ___ Spine

7th   ___ Hips

Good. We will come back to that in a few minutes.

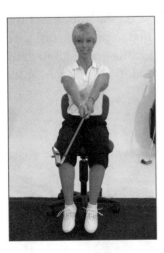

Next I would like you to sit in a swivel chair with a golf club in hand and your feet off the ground. ◀

Start with your feet off the ground and the golf club waist high, and make a backswing. ▶

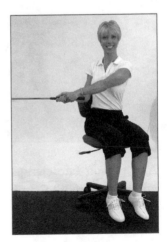

Which way did the swivel chair move? Clockwise or counterclockwise?

Try it again.

Sure enough, when you attempt to move the club in that sequence—clubhead first—you end up doing quite a bit of damage to your golf swing and your body. Let's take a closer look.

From the video, the sequence to your takeaway was most likely:

1st   Clubhead

2nd   Shaft

3rd   Hands

4th   Arms

5th   Shoulders

6th   Spine

7th   Hips

You will notice on the swivel chair that when the clubhead goes first, your body wants to turn counterclockwise. Yet the club needs to travel in the other direction.

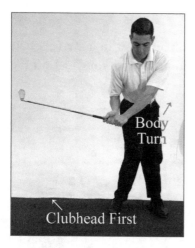

Body Turn

Clubhead First

This traps your spine in the middle and creates undue stress on the muscles of the back. So much so, that to ease this pressure your feet will release the ground and your balance will start to shift off center in order to compensate. ◄

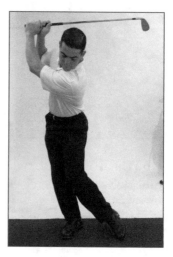

Any person knowledgeable about the spine will tell you that the upper spine doesn't turn more than twenty-five to thirty degrees, and the lower spine may give a bit, but it too is not designed to twist more than five degrees. ▶

Takeback Drill I

In order to create the safest and most powerful backswing, take a seat back on the swivel chair with your feet off of the ground and put the clubhead in your hands. Have the grip touching the ground, centered in front of you. ▶

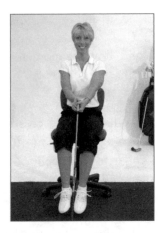

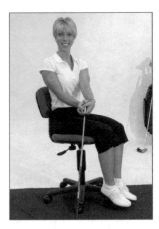

Point the shaft at your belly button in the dead center of your body. Gently apply force through the shaft straight into the ground. Did you turn? If the shaft is dead center, you will notice there is no turn in either direction. Continue to apply that force and move your hands slightly forward of center. ◀

Q. Did you turn? Which way?　A.

Now move your hands slightly back of center.

Q. Did you turn? Which way?　A.

Continue to move the hands a few inches forward of center and a few inches back of center in order to get the feel of this connection between the hands and the hips. Do this ten times. ▶

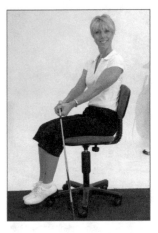

Takeback Drill II

Repeat Drill I with each hand individually, ten times each. This time, allow the club to fling on up as you spin around. Pay close attention to how the momentum of the club pivots the body.

Takeback Drill III

Stand up and repeat Drills I and II, ten times each. Notice how the momentum of the club pivots your body.

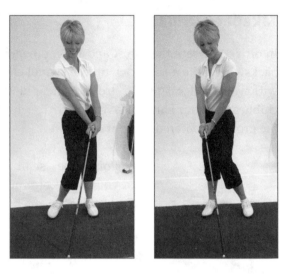

What we are creating here is a powerful machine similar to a propeller on a plane. Back in the early days of aviation, the crewmembers on the tarmac had to hand start the propeller in order to kick start the engine on the inside.

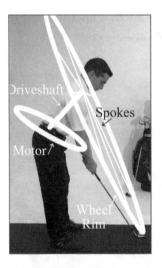

Looking at the illustration on the left, the clubhead would be at the tip of the propeller blade, the shaft the blade itself, and the center of the rotor similar to where the shoulders meet at the base of the neck. The driveshaft would coincide with the spine and lead to the engine, the hips. ◄

As you saw in your baseline video earlier, sequentially the clubhead was moving the hands, arms, shoulders, spine and then the hips, wrapping your shoulders against your feet and crushing your spine in the middle. ▶

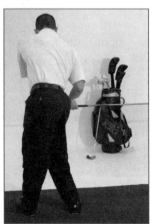

Technological advances in aviation now allow the pilot to push a button to start the engine, which turns the drive shaft to spin the propellers. Your golf swing should benefit from the same type of sequence.

By sitting on the swivel chair, you learned that the hips move in response to the hand action. When the hands move, they create the momentum necessary to move the hips.

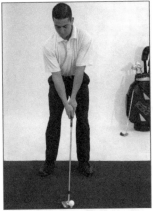

This momentum turns the hips, creating so much momentum that the clubhead and shaft hinge the wrists and load the club at top of the backswing.

This correct sequence loads your swing powerfully and without strain on the back because the hips are turning against your feet and the ground, and the club loads against your shoulders, all effortlessly with power.

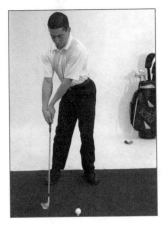

This action is similar to that of cracking a whip. If you were to crack a whip, which part of the whip would go first: the handle or the tip? Obviously, because of the slack of the whip, the tip could never go first. The handle must move first.

The same is true in your golf swing. Never think of the shaft as one solid piece, instead let it sling back like a brick on the end of a string, moving the clubhead last.

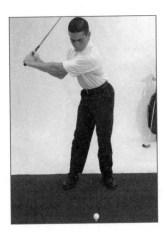

Having this viewpoint will enable you to remove the tension in the swing and attain a soft, free-flowing, slinging backswing that will be fully loaded to explode with power in the downswing!

Let's continue doing some more drills in order to ingrain this concept into your body.

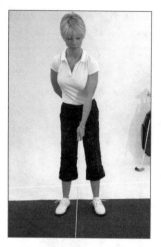

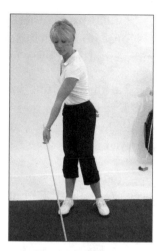

Takeback Drill IV

With the yardstick in your left hand, take your stance with your right arm placed behind you. ◄

Gently move your left hand straight back, leaving the tip of the yardstick where it is. ▸

This movement of the left hand will turn your hips clockwise, which in turn will release the tip of the yardstick. ◄

Do this with some speed, and as the tip of the stick moves, really make it drag and create some noise in the first fifteen inches going back. ▸

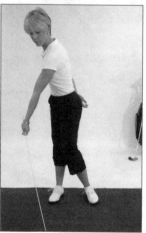

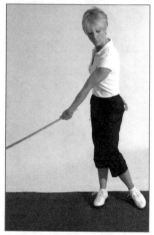

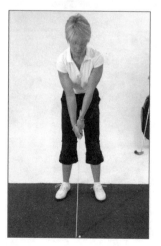

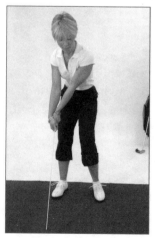

Repeat this drill five times. Add the right hand to the yardstick and repeat the drill five additional times. ◄

Make note that because of the very light weight of the yardstick it will be difficult to create the momentum necessary to complete a backswing; this is normal. When you eventually add the heavy club, there will be no problem getting the club back with momentum.

Now take the golf club in the left hand only. The additional weight should really be noticeable as you sling the handle back first. This is followed by the hip turn, which will in turn move the clubhead last.

Repeat this drill five times.

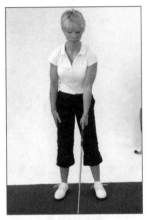
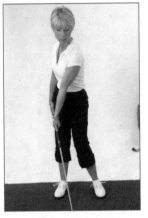
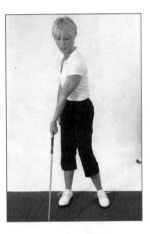

It's time to add the right hand and focus on
hands first,   hips second,   and clubhead third.

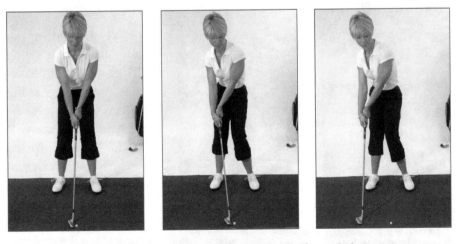

Just make backswings when doing these drills and do not attempt to swing through. By focusing on the backswing, your attention, rightfully so, is on something other than hitting the ball! Hitting a ball or making the downswing motion at this juncture would only set one up for a loss. Be diligent, not glib—do the drills as indicated, and you will be rewarded with the ultimate backswing built for power.

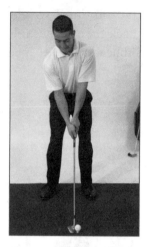

Now let's look at the start of your swing again. If you were to start your hands in the middle of your stance, opposite your zipper, and move your hands back, you would create X amount of momentum for the backswing. ◄

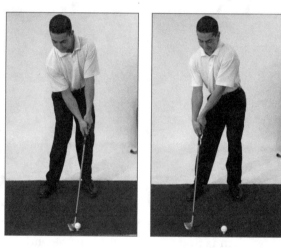

But by adding a forward press, you can create X amount of momentum plus distance traveled. ▸

Takeback Drill V

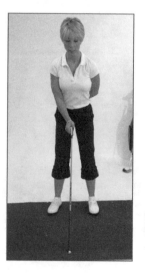

Think of a child trying to get started on a swing set. They move a little forward in order to get going backwards. It's the same thing here. Take the golf club and turn it upside down. Placing the clubhead in your right hand, press forward and move the hand forward of your belt buckle, allowing the hips to slightly turn counterclockwise.

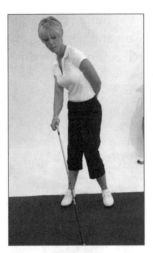

From there, move the hand back, allowing the hips to turn clockwise. This movement will in turn release the tip of the club, initiating the takeback. With the addition of this forward press, the starting sequence is now complete and can be broken down into: ◄

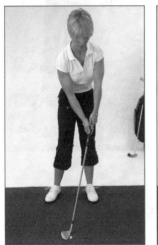 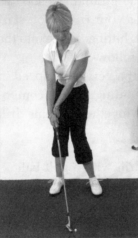 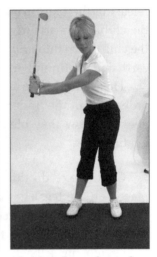

handle forward, hips turn counterclockwise,   handle backward, hips turn counterclockwise,   clubhead is released.

Change to the yardstick, and now with both hands on, drill this five times. Switch back to the club, and using both hands, drill this five times.

Do this drill as many times as you need until it is fluid and you have total certainty on the sequence of this chain reaction. Once you have achieved this, it is time to blend your start with what you learned in impact and follow-through.

Note: The golf swing, as we are laying it out here, is akin to the management of spinning plates. The golf swing has been broken down into its key components, and then each component has its appropriate drills laid out in their proper sequence. Each individual piece is like a spinning plate. You have a few plates you have to keep spinning as you learn another piece, but realize that it is not many plates in the end, and if each component is done correctly, it is quite manageable for the keen golfer.

BLENDING DRILL I

Position a tee in the ground. With both hands on the golf club, do just a slight forward press by moving the hands slightly forward of center, and let the hips be turned out of the way counter-clockwise. From there rebound off by moving the hands back, letting the hips turn clockwise, and releasing the club from the ground. As soon as the clubhead starts to pass your right foot, start the club down into impact, hitting the tee into the earth and continuing into follow-through.

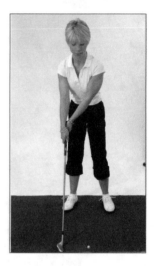

This should be done at a very slow speed in order to gain the understanding of each component and how they blend together. Do this drill ten times.

Continue to do this drill with a golf ball placed on the tee. The ball should not travel more than twenty feet in doing this exercise. If it does, you are doing this too fast, and/or taking too big a backswing. These are just miniature swings. Do this drill ten times.

Repeat these two drills for ten minutes on the first day.

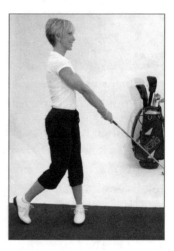

This is the end of the drills of Lesson Three. To gain the most from of this lesson, do the drills one time through the first day. Come back tomorrow and repeat the drills, this time twice through. Take the third day off. On the fourth day, do the drills three times through, bumping the numbers up threefold.

LESSON FOUR: THE CHANGE

The anatomy of control is the ability to start, change, and stop. There is no such thing as partial control, you either have it or you don't. If you start your car and change its location by driving around town, but you are unable to stop it, then you had no control over the car. The same is true in your golf swing. At this point, we've introduced you to the start of your swing with the takeback, and as far as the ball is concerned, impact is the end of the swing. With those two stable endpoints covered, it is time to introduce you to changing the direction of the club during the unloading phases of the backswing and downswing.

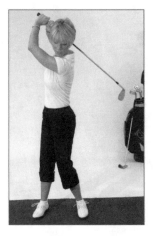

First let's talk about the backswing. With a golf club in hand, stand in front of a mirror and make the biggest back-swing you can make. Did your backswing look like this? ◄

Or like this? ▶

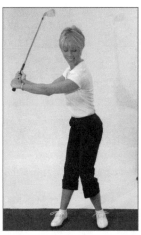

You'll notice I asked for a *back*swing, not an

upswing,   long swing,   forward swing,

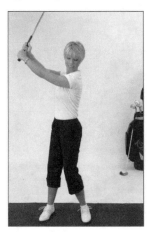

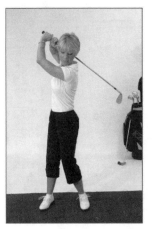

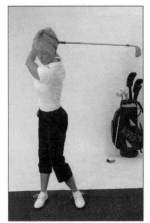

or anything else. By definition *back* is *back* away from the ball's flight of travel. Any backswing that takes the hands higher than chest to shoulder height starts to become inefficient.

Think about it. If I were to ask you to throw a ball, would you take the ball back,   up,   forward,

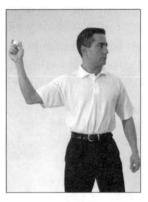
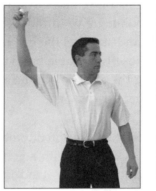
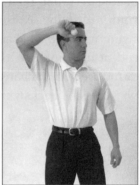

back to back,   and then unload it?

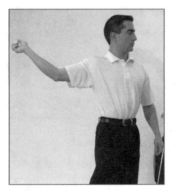
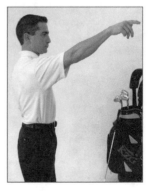

Or would you just take it back and throw it?

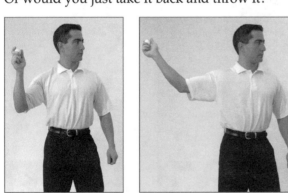

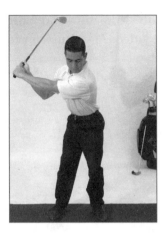

Any time you change direction of the golf club, you have to slow the club down, then stop and restart it. To maximize your energy transfer in golf, just load the club back and unload to the ball.

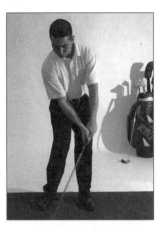

The following drills are going to show you how to achieve this powerful and compact *back*swing.

Change Drill I

Start by hitting a few full shots, using your hands forward, hips turn, handle back, hips turn, clubhead last takeaway. Get your video camera, and record a few swings. Where do your hands end up at the top of the backswing? Is there space between your hands and your head? Do your arms have extension at the end of your backswing?

After reviewing this footage, some of you

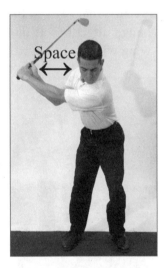

may already have a perfectly efficient backswing. To these people, I say well done, and you have permission to move on to the next section of the book. For all the rest, the following drill will bring you right up to the front of the class.

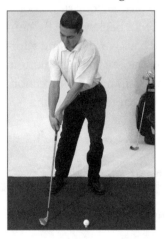

Again with the video recording, I want you to start your golf swing as indicated before, but this time really brush the turf loudly for the first fifteen inches (or where the club lines up opposite of your right foot) of the takeaway.

At which time I want you to change the club's direction and start down. Do this drill three times, then look at it on video. Ask yourself the following questions:

Q. Where did your golf swing actually change directions?

A.

Q. Were you able to change directions when you thought you did?

A.

Q. Did you think your swing still went that far back?

A.

Because of the momentum we created for you in the forward press and takeaway, there is no way you are going to be able to change club direction that early in the swing. The intention to change directions at that moment in your backswing will create a perfect *back*-backswing.

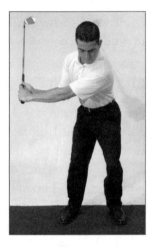

If you wait too long, you will miss this window of opportunity to harness the loading power of the shaft and, in effect, create an ill-desired long golf swing.

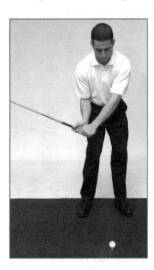

Hit a few more shots, keying in on starting down as soon as the club passes your right foot.

Remember, it is called a backswing. By definition, it must be swung backwards. Using a forward press to create the swinging motion, coupled with the early change of direction, ensures the backward direction for the club.

THE STARTDOWN

Now that we have discussed how to load your golf swing, the fun part begins—how to unload all of this stored energy!

Unloading the golf club is just like throwing a ball. By definition, a throw has two components. First, it must have an extension force, and second, it must have a release. One without the other is not a throw.

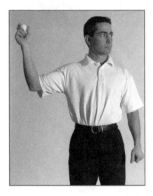
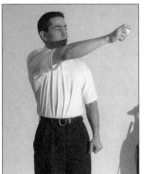
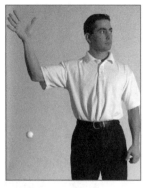

A directional force without a release is a balk, and a release without force behind it is a drop. The balance of these two components in golf is very natural if you extend your arms first, and then allow the body to release as a result of this extension.

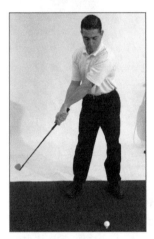
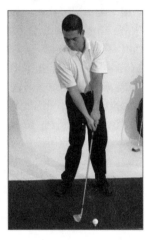

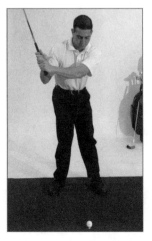
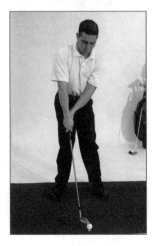

Be sure not to fall into the most common mistake in golf, which is to reverse these two components and try to release your body (turn) before you extend.

Here is another look from behind the ball.

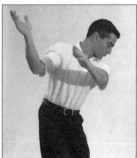
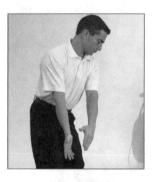
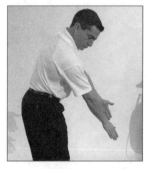

The simplicity of the startdown is that you are unloading the golf club toward the ball. This unloading requires an extension of both arms in the correct direction. The clubhead is directed using pressure against the proximal phalanx bone of the index finger down,

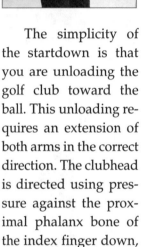
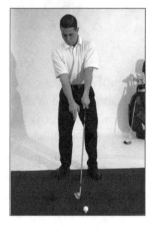

out, and slightly forward from where it is at the end of the backswing. With energy, this direction is called a vector force. Your effort to move the clubhead in this straight line to the golf ball will move the golf club in an arc.

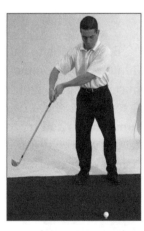
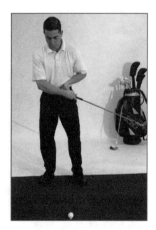

Never try to recreate the arc. Just focus on moving your finger on a straight line, and the club will travel in the appropriate arc to the ball.

Startdown Drill I

Place a golf ball on the ground, and with your left hand behind your back, move your right hand to the top of the backswing using your new forward press, and takeaway, and then fire your right index finger to the golf ball. Make sure your right index finger is pointing at the ball. Do this five times.

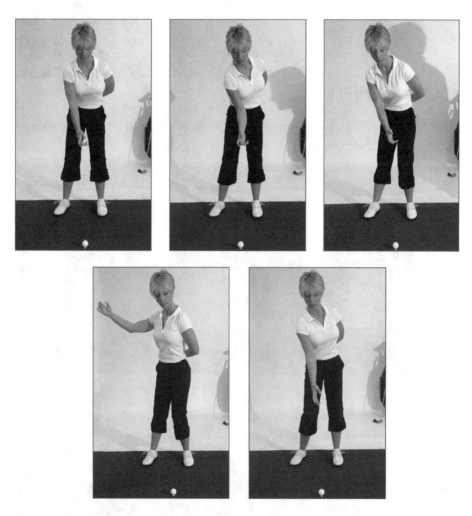

Startdown Drill II

Repeat the action in Drill I, and then continue to extend the right index finger to the ball, turning the body through and into the follow-through.

At the end of this drill, your body should be in the same alignment as you were on completion of the exercise in Follow-through Drill I (see page 257). Do this five times. ▸

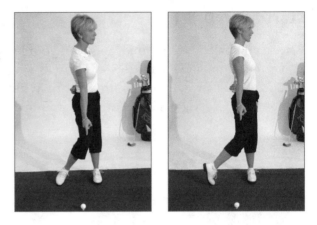

Startdown Drill III

Now hold a golf ball in your right hand and repeat Drill I, this time throwing the ball at the ball on the ground. ▾

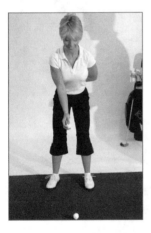
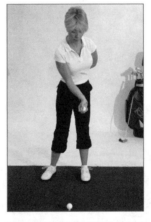
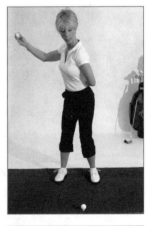

Make sure you have enough room on the opposite side of the ball if you are indoors. You will notice that the direction you throw the ball is the down, out, and slightly forward vector force as described earlier. Do this five times. ▸

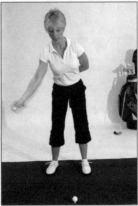
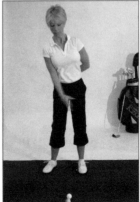

Startdown Drill IV

Grip the tennis racquet, and using your forward press and takeaway, ▼

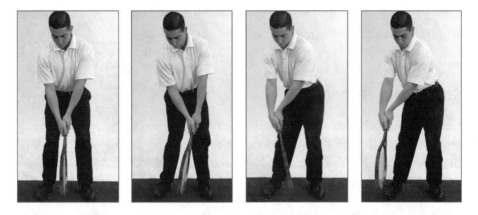

take it to the top of the backswing. Start the racquet down toward the ground without the body turning. ▶

The shaft at this point will be inline with the left arm and left shoulder, with the face of the racquet pointing at the golf ball. From this position, keep the

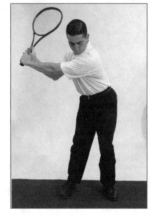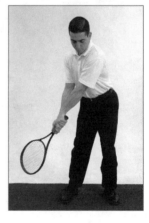

structured alignment of the racquet against your left arm and move the racquet toward the ball. ◀

You will notice that this extension out toward the ball rotates the body to release, and thus square up, the face for impact. ▶

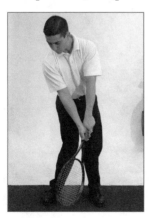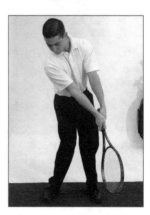

Continue this extension against the racquet and allow the body to release all the way through, into the follow-through position. ▸

The racquet should be in alignment with your left arm all the way up to your left shoulder. Do this five times.

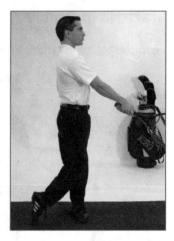

Startdown Drill V

Grip the golf club down by the hosel (left), and take it to the top of the backswing (middle). Start the club down toward the ground without the body turning (right).

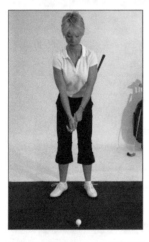
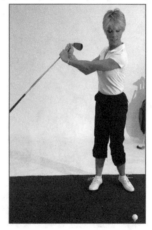
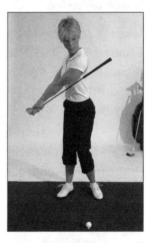

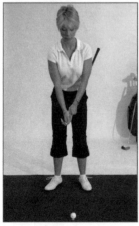

The shaft at this point will be inline with the left arm and left shoulder, with the leading edge of the golf club pointing at the golf ball. Bring the club back to the top of your backswing and repeat.

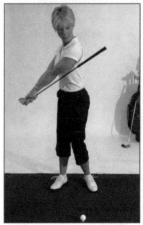

Bring the club back to the top of the backswing a third time, and this time allow the body to release on through as the effect of this third extension—all the way through into the follow-through position. The shaft should be in alignment with your left arm all the way up to your left shoulder. Do this five times. ▸

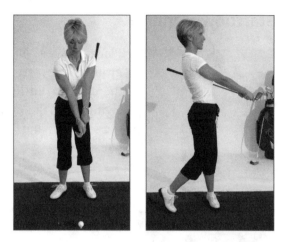

Startdown Drill VI

Repeat Drill V, this time holding the shaft at the midpoint. Do this five times.

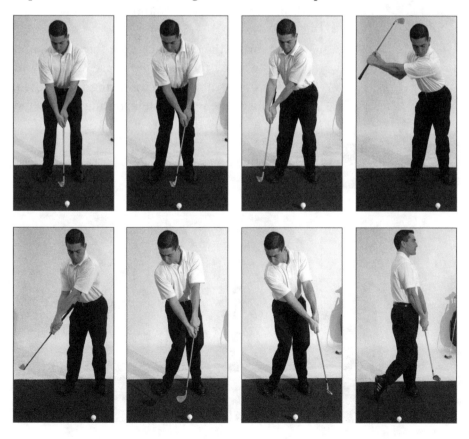

Startdown Drill VII

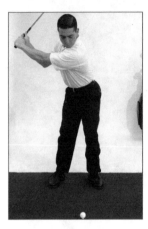

Place a tee in the ground and, gripping the club at full length, swing it to the end of the backswing and pause. ◀

Start the club down to the ground without the body turning. ▶

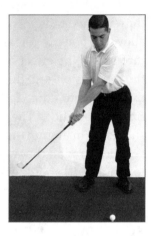

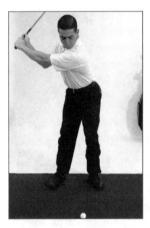

Bring the club back up and repeat. ◀

Again, bring the club back up a third time, and this time allow the body to release on this third effort as a result of the club being fired down, swinging all the way through, hitting the tee, and ending at follow-through. ▼

Do this five times.

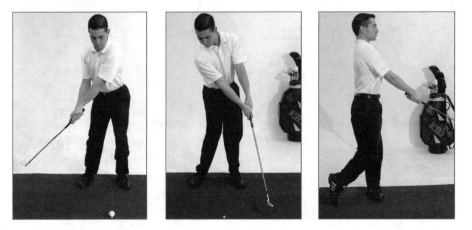

Startdown Drill VIII

Now it is time to just hit the tee. All of your efforts and your drilling are about to pay off. Sling the clubhead back, and extend the clubhead to the tee, having the body release as the effect of your extension.

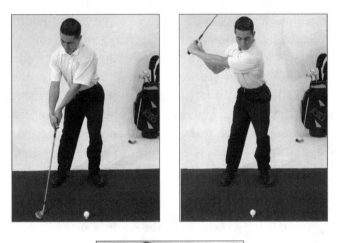

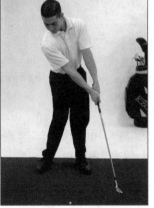

Do this ten times.

Cycle through the drills in Lesson Four the first day and twice the following day. On the third day, you should be ready to hit the practice range.

THE PRACTICE RANGE

At this point you should be getting a good feel for how the sequence of the startdown occurs. The extension of the clubhead toward the ball causes the release of the body. Now it is time to start blending all of the components you have learned thus far and hitting balls at a practice range, though we will limit your shots to a maximum of seventy-five yards to start, as we have yet to give you the final component of the swing—the finish.

You will only need one club to start with—a sand wedge, pitching wedge, or nine-iron will be sufficient. When you arrive at the range, get yourself a bucket of fifty balls or so (you really don't need the mega-jumbo bucket), and find a secluded, quiet spot near one of the ends where you can

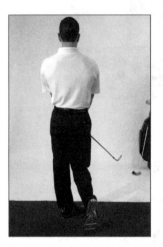

focus in peace and not be distracted. Take a few practice swings to loosen up those muscles, then take a few more focused practice swings on your sequence. Strike the rubber tee if you are hitting off of Astroturf mats, or place your own tee in the ground if you are hitting off of real grass. Focus on your forward-press take-away, slinging the club back, handle—hips—handle—hips—clubhead last, and starting down with the clubhead extending toward the ball first, allowing the body to release as the effect. Take five practice swings hitting the tee. Then tee up a ball, and hit it using the same action.

Take five more practice swings, hitting the tee each time (start over if you don't get five in a row), and hit another golf ball. Once you accomplish that with confidence, take four practice swings, and hit two balls. Then three and three, two and four, and finally down to one and five. Finish off by hitting ten shots in a row with confidence.

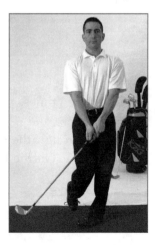

At the end of these shots your body will be in alignment as it was in the follow-through: club-head low, hands and arms extended, spine straight, head vertical on top of the neck with eyes level, and right foot fully released on its toes with the bottom of the right shoe facing back.

Push versus Pull: The Great Golfing Debate

Golf instruction has long maintained that the golf swing is a pulling motion. New technologies have brilliantly countered this old way of thinking and destroyed it. Yet interestingly enough, why has the traditional viewpoint not changed? Let's take a closer look and bring to the forefront the truth.

Muscles in the human body work by contraction. Your elbow folds as your bicep muscle shortens. Your arm extends as your triceps contract. This is indisputable.

Now, if you think past what the muscles do and focus on the end product, you would see that when you extend your arms away from your torso, this is a pushing motion. When you bring something closer to your torso you are pulling it in.

At impact you want to have your arms extending out to the ball.

Any type of extension, therefore, is a pushing action. Conversely, if you were to try to pull on the club successfully, you should never make contact with the ball. Your arms would be bringing the club up and toward your torso.

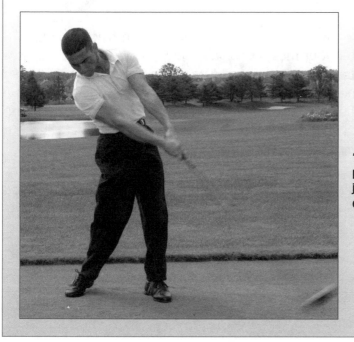

"There's no pulling here—just pure extension!"

What about clubhead throwaway, you ask? Don't you have to delay the hit and create a late-hit angle?

Good questions. The argument is never do you have to delay the hit, the delayed hit, or late-hit angle, is created automatically when you attempt to extend your arms toward the ball. Clubhead throwaway is created when you extend you arms in a direction other than toward the golf ball.

Consider this. A downswing lasts about .18 of a second, on the first .16 of a second you see the delayed hit/late hit angle. There is no possible way that even the best touring professional would be able to pull on the handle of the club for the first .16 of a second and then extend the last .02 of a second. *Impossible!* The clubface would be stuck wide open, and you would slice it. Hmmm, maybe that's why one slices?

Any extending motion at speed looks like a pulling motion. Whether it is a punch in a boxing ring, a cast of a fishing rod, a hit with baseball bat, or shooting a basketball, Newton's first law of motion still applies! The heavy weighted object in a golf swing (the clubhead) wants to continue traveling backwards even though you want to start down. By the time you notice the startdown, your clubhead has either 1) slowed down, 2) stopped, 3) or changed directions, and then 4) accelerated on the newly instructed path. All you did was tell your muscles to start down, while the clubhead is going off of its previously received data of "go back," and the differential outcome is a late-hit angle. Now, the harder you attempt to hit the ball, the more the clubhead will resist and create more of a late-hit angle, and the farther the ball will go.

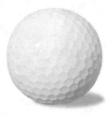

LESSON FIVE: SETUP AND FINISH

Most traditional golf instruction focuses the first lesson on getting the student the perfect grip and stance. Remember that "traditional" golf instruction doesn't work. That's why now that we are nearing the end of your Atomic Golf instruction it is time we discuss these important components.

Let us ask you this: if you had the perfect grip and stance, and were aimed perfectly at the flag, but you had agreed to the false belief that you had to swing up to make the ball go into the air, would it make a difference how you held the club? Or where you stood? Of course not! In fact, you would adjust your grip, stance, and aim in order to accommodate this false belief!

The grip and stance have their correct time and place of introduction in the Atomic Golf System, and that is once the student either is in need of the right grip because they have no information on the grip, or once they understand that what they have to do with the club makes it necessary to hold it in an optimal position.

The Grip

When gripping the club, hold it in your left hand as you would hold a hammer. That is, under the heel pad of the hand and not the thumb pad!

The wrist will be on top of the club with the heel pad on top of the grip —not in front of the grip, or with the palm facing down at the grip.

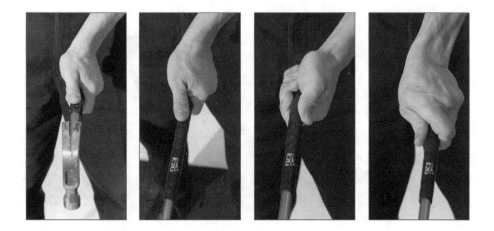

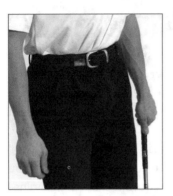

The best place to apply the grip is here, ◄

opposite the left heel, with your hand applying pressure behind you. ▶

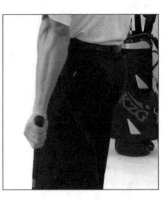

In fact, you can practice hammering the sole of the club against the

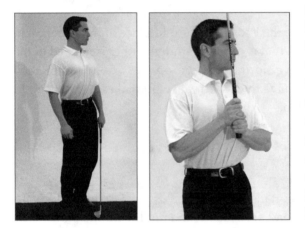

ground for confirmation that your left hand is perfectly positioned. Double-check when you grip the club that the leading edge of the clubface is at a right angle to your chosen target. (left) Now, to assemble the right hand, swing the left hand up in front of you at chest height. (right)

You will notice the base of the lifeline of your right hand is perfectly made to join the second knuckle up from your left thumbnail, also called the metacarpophalangeal joint of the thumb.

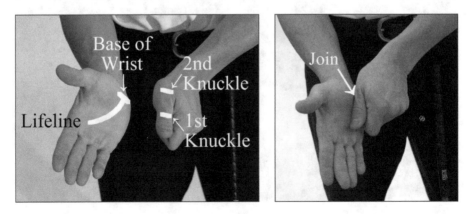

From there, just wrap your fingers around the club.

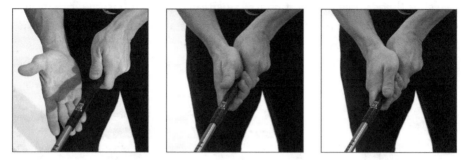

Apply these two primary alignments of the grip and you will never again have to worry about your grip.

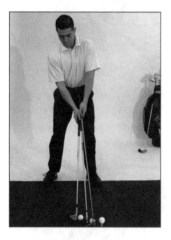

Ball Position

Now that you have your grip solid, for all standard shots, place the golf ball in the first third of your stance.

With the longer clubs, you will position the ball a little closer to the left foot, and position it a little closer to the center of your stance with the shorter clubs. Only play the ball in the center third or back third of your stance if you are attempting to play some sort of specialty shot.

Stance

The proper stance starts out with your heels underneath your hip joints, both feet slightly turned out, and your knees unlocked—not bent or straight. A shaft placed across the line of your toes should parallel where you would like the ball to finish.

When you bring your

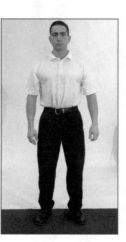
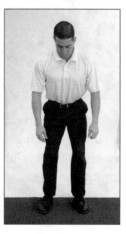

hands together, your right shoulder will drop and your left shoulder will rise slightly because the right hand's position on the club is lower than that of the left hand. This will create just the right amount of tilt in the spine. This is the proper posture for golf.

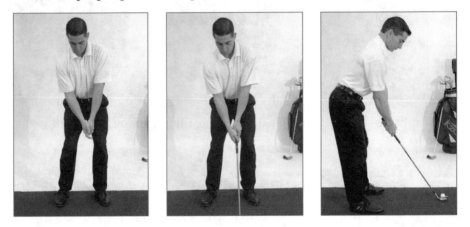

These three components of grip, ball position, and stance can be married together to form a preshot routine. When you get to play on the golf course, and it's your turn to hit, you will first determine which club you are going to hit with, take it out of the bag, and start your preshot routine:

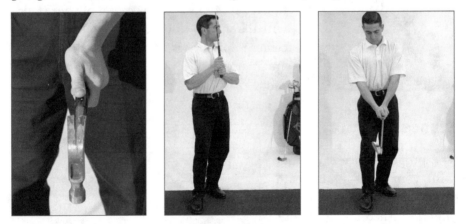

Stand to the side of the golf ball, and put your left hand on the club as if you are holding a hammer. (left)

Swing the club up in front of you and assemble the right hand. (middle)

Lower the club to waist height to double-check your grip with the club-face's leading edge. (right)

Take a step with your right foot to line up the clubface to the ball and target. (left)

Position your left foot forward for your ball placement. (middle)

Position your right foot back for balance. (right)

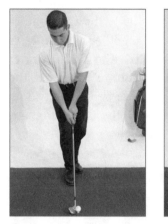 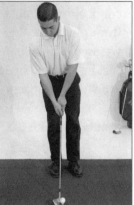 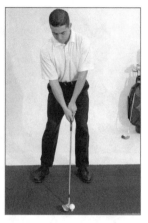

Take a final look at the flag . . .

. . . and enjoy whacking the heck out of it!

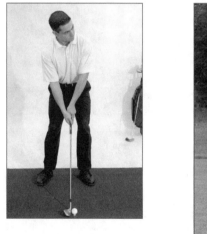 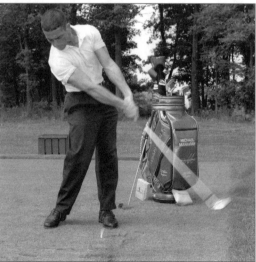

The steps in the setup, once learned, should be applied to every shot when you play golf. When you are practicing, you should make it second nature to apply your grip and stance in this standard way.

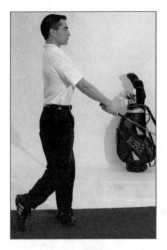

The Finish

It is time to finish your golf swing. As you have learned by now, when you add speed to your golf swing, the arms no longer maintain that connection against the body in the follow-through, but rather rise together as a unit. As we mentioned before, like the figure skater turning on ice, the faster you turn the more the arms want to rise. As you hit a golf shot, allow the arms to raise up naturally as the momentum takes them up. ◄

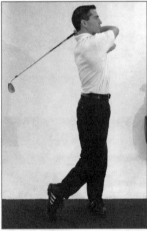

Do not force the arms up, just gently allow them to go where they want to, up and over the left shoulder. ◄

The elbows will fold first, followed by the wrists. ▶

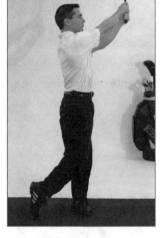

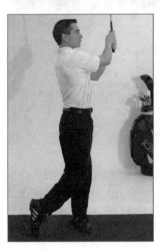

From there, allow them to recoil by un-folding the elbows first and the wrists second. ◄

From here, gently let the club slide down into your fingers ▶

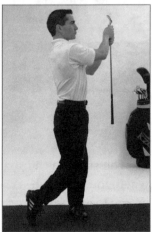

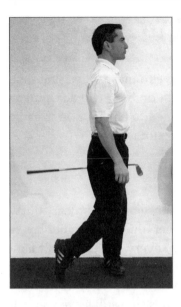

and into your left hand, followed by your arms dangling by your sides with the club in your left hand. ◀

This finish indicates how well you have performed every prior action. You will be in a relaxed, balanced position, watching the ball fly toward your intended target. It is difficult to hit a good shot and not finish, and it's rare to ever see a bad shot with a finish. Stand proud on every shot and make a solid finish, enjoying that ball fly toward your intended target.

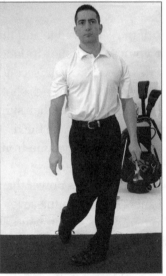

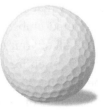

LESSON SIX: PRACTICE AND WARM-UP

Whenever you go to the driving range, you have to make a decision first: are you there to warm up or practice? Trying to do both will accomplish nothing! The following two routines are designed to enhance your game whether you are there for practice or to warm up for a round.

The Warm up

Before you go out and play a round of golf, allot yourself at least thirty minutes to arrive at the golf club and soak in everything the facility has to offer you. I understand that in the real world, every round of golf isn't played like a Sunday afternoon at a Major. But thirty minutes is plenty of time to head to the practice tee, get fifteen minutes of prep time in, head over to the putting/chipping green for ten minutes, and still leave yourself five minutes to get ready to play.

In those fifteen minutes at the range, start with the sand wedge and hit your first shot twenty feet in front of you. Hit your second shot to land where the first one ended up. Hit your third shot to land where your second shot landed. Repeat this for five shots, expanding the distance on each shot. By the fifth shot of this sequence, you should be hitting a full shot. Then skip over your pitching wedge and hit your nine-iron for five shots, with the first shot landing where your last sand wedge finished. Expand on the nine-iron, hitting each shot to land at the distance the previous shot finished.

You have now gradually hit ten shots, each with a little more power than the previous shot. Continue now to hit four full shots each with the seven-iron and five-iron; two shots with either your three-iron or a seven-wood, if you carry one of these new hybrid clubs; three shots with your main fairway wood; and follow it with five shots with your driver. Now you should be fully warmed up. Next go back to your seven-iron and hit four shots, simulating golf-course conditions. Focus on where you want the ball to end up, take your grip and stance, and enjoy that strike! You have gone through your bag, hitting all of the odd-numbered clubs. Next time you warm up, start with your pitching wedge and hit all of your even-numbered clubs; this way you will ensure an even wear on your entire set of clubs.

Now let's head over to the putting green. Take three golf balls and line them up one, two, and three feet away on the same line.

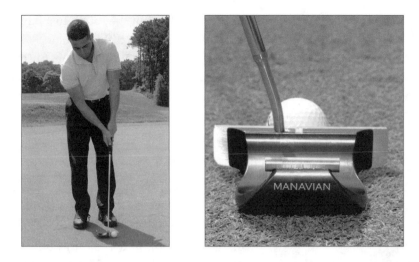

Knock each one in, and repeat this action from all four sides of the hole—north, south, east, and west. This way you ensure that you are warming up by hitting putts that break with a different angle—right to left, left to right, uphill, and downhill.

Once you have hit those twelve putts, putt three balls from four feet away, this time from the in-between angles: northeast, southwest, northwest, and southeast.

Your only focus here is to warm up; as a final product, you get the correct speed of the greens for that day. By hitting putts from these eight different directions, you will get an idea of how true the greens will be rolling that day.

Move over to the fringe and hit three chips with your seven-iron to a flag, and then hit three more chips in a different direction.

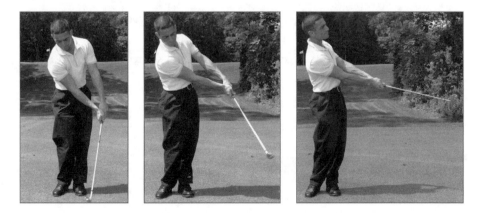

Take your sand wedge and hit three shots from the rough to a flag, and then hit three more shots from a different angle to a different flag.

At this time, you are ready to go out and play. Warming up is just warming up. Done properly, it will put you in the correct frame of mind and will give you some excellent data on the day's course conditions that you can use for when you are playing.

Practicing

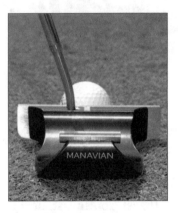

On the days you are not playing golf, or after a round of golf if you decide you would like to practice your golf swing, go back to the drills in this book and cycle through them. Alternatively, if you would like to practice hitting shots *with* your swing, I will recommend the following routine for the practice range. Practicing your swing and practicing hitting shots are two entirely different items. Beginners and intermediate players should stick to practicing their swings with the drills. Once you begin progressing, go ahead and start introducing the following practice routine for your golf shots:

Day 1: Short irons, long irons

Day 2: Medium irons, fairway woods, driver

Drills Day I

Clubs: Short irons, lob wedge, sand wedge, pitching wedge, nine-iron, and eight-iron

Set up three balls at four different stations. Cycle through the following shots three times:

Station 1   Low shots

Station 2   High shots

Station 3   Hard shots

Station 4   Standard shots

Clubs: Long irons (2, 3, 4)

Set up three balls at five different stations. Cycle through the following shots three times:

Station 1 Low shots (hit off of a tee with the two-iron)

Station 2 Fades

Station 3 Draws

Station 4 Hard shots

Station 5 Standard shots

Drills Day II

Clubs: Medium irons (5, 6, 7)

Set up three balls at five different stations. Cycle through the following shots three times:

Station 1 Low shots (hit off of a tee)

Station 2 Fades

Station 3 Draws

Station 4 Hard shots

Station 5 Standard shots

Clubs: Fairway woods (5 wood, 3 wood, hybrids)

Set up three balls at five different stations. Cycle through the following shots three times:

Station 1 Hit out of the rough

Station 2 Fades

Station 3 Draws

Station 4 Hard off of fairway

Station 5 Standard tee shots

Club: Driver

Set up three balls at five different stations. Cycle through the following shots three times:

Station 1   Hit off of the fairway

Station 2   Fade off the tee

Station 3   Draw off the tee

Station 4   Hard off the tee

Station 5   Standard shot off the tee

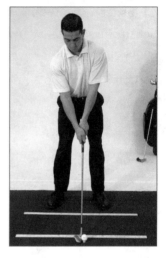

Note on curving the ball: thus far we have shown you only how to hit standard shots. ▶

To curve the ball right to left, or left to right, simply point the clubface where you would like the ball to end up, and turn your body parallel to where you would like the ball to start. ▼

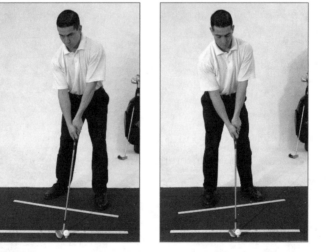

On the practice tee, you may place the yardstick or a golf club on your toe line to aid you as an alignment guide, as shown in the pictures.

The Importance of Properly Fit Golf Clubs

*N*ow that you have developed your golf swing, you want to be able to demonstrate this knowledge using golf clubs that reward your technique. The perfect club for you is one that was put together specifically for your swing. As we discussed earlier, everyone's golf swing is as unique to them as a fingerprint. Therefore, no two people should play with the same clubs—never mind buying the same set off the rack. But as you realize by now, the golf industry isn't going to keep making profits if your set of clubs fit you appropriately. You are now responsible for finding yourself a custom clubfitter near you that will be able to take your swing and build clubs or modify your existing clubs to match your swing. For a list of clubfitters, see page 321.

THE PURPOSE OF PROPERLY FIT GOLF CLUBS

The purpose of properly fit golf clubs is to reward your intended swing. If we as instructors ask you to make a certain motion with the golf club, and the ball keeps going offline, you will naturally stop making that motion and start to make a different motion in order to make the ball go straight. Note the chart on page 302.

A shot with a seven-iron that is two degrees off will miss the target by approximately 10.5 feet from 150 yards. Never mind a club that is eight or ten degrees off, which can send a ball offline by more than fifty feet! Ask any clubfitter; this is more common than one would think.

Having this information now is like a double-edged sword; it would be a violation of your integrity not to get clubs that match your swing!

THE EFFECT ON ACCURACY WITH THE WRONG LIE ANGLE

		Deviation from Target					Directional Displacement				
CLUB	YARDAGE	2°	4°	6°	8°	10°	2°	4°	6°	8°	10°
2	200	0.61°	1.22°	1.83°	2.44°	3.04°	6.4'	12.8'	19.2'	25.5'	31.9'
3	190	0.73°	1.45°	2.18°	2.90°	3.62°	7.2'	14.5'	21.7'	28.9'	36.0'
4	180	0.85°	1.70°	2.54°	3.38°	4.22°	8.0'	16.0'	24.0'	31.9'	39.8'
5	170	0.98°	1.95°	2.92°	3.88°	4.82°	8.7'	17.4'	26.0'	34.6'	43.2'
6	160	1.15°	2.31°	3.45°	4.59°	5.73°	9.7'	19.3'	29.0'	38.6'	48.1'
7	150	1.35°	2.69°	4.03°	5.36°	6.68°	10.6'	21.1'	31.7'	42.2'	52.7'
8	140	1.56°	3.12°	4.67°	6.21°	7.73°	11.5'	22.9'	34.3'	45.7'	57.0'
9	130	1.80°	3.59°	5.38°	7.14°	8.89°	12.3'	24.5'	36.7'	48.9'	61.0'
PW	120	2.07°	4.13°	6.18°	8.20°	10.19°	13.0'	26.0'	39.0'	51.9'	64.7'
GW	110	2.38°	4.75°	7.10°	9.42°	11.69°	13.7'	27.4'	41.1'	54.7'	68.3'
SW	100	2.85°	5.69°	8.49°	11.24	13.93°	15.0'	29.9'	44.8'	59.6'	74.4'

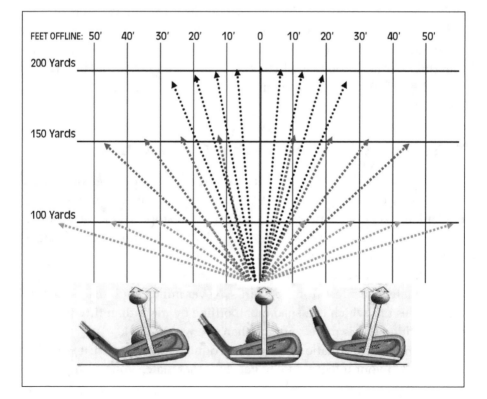

This is just one example of what custom-fitting covers. A full text could be written on the fine-tuning aspect and idiosyncrasies of custom-fitting. That is not the intention of this text. As authors, we merely want to show some common pitfalls to avoid when purchasing clubs and provide pertinent questions to ask in order to be optimally fit.

YOUR SET MAKEUP

When getting fit, you must take into consideration the following options: your set makeup—how many clubs do you need? If you are a beginner, start with a partial set of five to six clubs and gain mastery over those. A five-wood for tee shots, a seven-iron, nine-iron, and sand wedge for the irons, and a putter is a fine starter set. When you start to see a demand for a club that you don't have, you can always fill it in later.

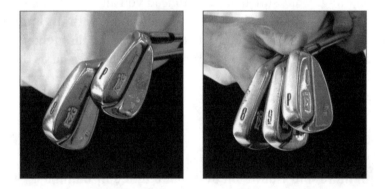

The set makeup for more advanced players has different requirements. Advanced players should really have a variety of different clubs so they can choose an optimal set for certain courses and different conditions. Their set should contain an extra fairway wood or a hybrid club instead of a two- or three-iron, and the right wedge combinations. Some courses will require a gap wedge or a lob wedge, in addition to your pitching and sand wedges.

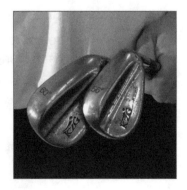

Just make sure that when you step on the first tee you have no more than the maximum allowable clubs of fourteen.

SHAFTS

The shaft is hands down by far the most important part of the golf club. It is in the end what loads and unloads your energy and transfers it to the ball. The shaft's flexibility, material, wall thickness, pattern, length, and location of its spine all contribute to having the shaft work best for you. If nothing else, you should seek a fitter that is experienced in shaft alignment. This will optimize each shaft within your set to load and unload to its full capacity.

CLUBHEADS

Manufacturers would like for you to believe that their current clubhead design is the latest and greatest thing since sliced bread. But in fact, the only significant feature they can change that affects the club's performance is the weighting. Make sure that the clubhead you and your fitter select has a center of gravity that fits your desired ball flight, with the appropriate amount of offset, and an appropriate loft progression throughout the set. There are many other important features of a clubhead as far as the finish, materials, different grinds, and aesthetic features that your experienced clubfitter can walk you through.

DID YOU KNOW?
Helpful Hints and Tidbits on Golf Clubs and Golf Swings

- The number one problem in golf is trying to swing up into the air.

- Trying to hit the ball "straight" will produce a slice.

- Divots come after the ball is contacted by the club.

- Wedges are the shortest clubs, yet they are the heaviest clubs, and the driver is the longest and lightest.

- The word *golf* derives from the Scottish word *gawf* or *gowff*, which means to strike with the open hand.

- If your clubs are off even by two degrees in lie angle, the resulting one hundred-yard shot from a sand wedge can be off as much as fifteen feet!

GRIP SIZE AND COMPOSITION

Choosing the right grip is crucial as that is the only part of the club you actually have contact with. The size of the grip's circumference is based on the length of your fingers. You want to be able to have a firm hold on the club with your fingers wrapped around the grip. A grip that is too large will inhibit the proper hand action through the shot, and one that is too small will have your fingers digging into your palm. Grips today come in a wide variety of compositions. It is a matter of personal preference which material you choose. With the advancements in technology over the years, manufacturers have produced wonderful grips that are made out of leather, rubber, and other synthetic materials.

BALLS

Choosing the right ball for your game involves finding the appropriate balance of a few variables. The most important variable is to find a ball that matches your driver in order to maximize your launch angle at impact, the spin rate, and initial ball velocity. Simply put, a ball that launches high, spins at a low rate, and moves fast will go the furthest and straightest under most conditions. An average golfer can easily gain twenty yards just

- A golfer with a twelve-degree launch angle, swinging at 90 mph under fairly normal conditions, could gain an additional nine yards of carry by going from a driver with nine degrees of loft to one with thirteen degrees.

- A golfer is allowed to carry a maximum of fourteen clubs per round. Though most amateurs would do considerably better by taking out half of their irons.

- The term *caddie* comes from the French word *cadet* pronounced cad-day.

- The first sand wedge was invented by the prominent American golfer Gene Sarazen, who soldered lead to the back of his niblick, which helped him to win the 1932 British Open.

- All golf-swing related injuries occur by pulling on the club.

by having a ball fitting that optimizes their driver. There are other factors you want to look at besides just hitting it far off the tee, and these have to do with how the ball feels and reacts around the green for your short shots, as well as its balance of spin with the angle of descent for your approach shots. Any good clubfitter will have a device called a launch monitor that will be able to calculate all of your ball flight data and make the appropriate recommendations.

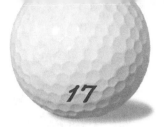

17

Playing Golf:
The Final Atomic Product

*O*ur goal is that by the end of this book you will be well on your way to playing great golf. In this final chapter we will show you how to:

1. **Look and assess the situation confronting you.** Ask yourself: where is my ball located, and where do I want to hit this ball? What are my shot conditions? Where is the wind coming from? How hard is it blowing? How much fairway or green is there available in the area I want to hit the ball?

2. **Choose the appropriate shot to play.** What shot will get me to my desired location?

3. **Affix your intention on the task.** Focus your mind on making that intention a reality in the physical universe.

4. **Execute the play.** Step up to the ball and hit it.

5. **Statistically assess the result.** Did your ball end up where you intended it to go? Yes or no?

Imagine that you are approaching the first tee. You've warmed up as we have shown you and are ready to go and play golf. It's now your turn to hit. You step up to the tee markers and are faced with a golf hole. Believe it or not, some golfers have actually gotten sick to their stomach just by doing this much! At this moment, there are countless distractions waiting to rob you of your intention. Some are specifically crafted by the golf course architect in the form of hazards and challenges, others by the people you're about to play golf with. Instead of getting caught up in these very tempting distractions, utilize the above five steps.

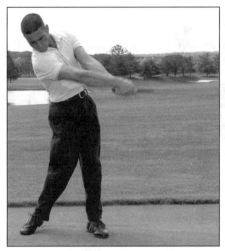

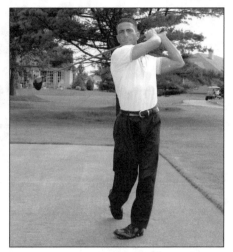

Power . . .   . . . and control:
                                              the product of Atomic Golf.

In this scenario, let's say that the ball is on the tee, and a shot of 250 yards down the middle will do. The wind is blowing from the right at a low rate, so you will aim slightly right of center in order for the wind to push it back. Good! Now convert what that means to what you can do.

Converting your situation to a shot is fairly simple and is something that will improve as you become more familiar with your golf game. In this case, it requires the use of a driver with a standard swing, nothing fancy. Take a practice swing if you like to get the idea of what a 250-yard standard driver shot takes to produce.

Before you step up to the ball to execute your shot, you need to clarify what your intention is for the golf ball. For this shot, putting the ball into the fairway is your sole intention.

Now with a clear-cut intention, step up from the side of the ball to execute your shot and execute it.

After the shot has landed and stopped, ask yourself, is that where you intended the ball to go? If so, then make a note of it; if not, make note of that as well.

At the end of the round, all we are concerned about is adding up the total amount of intended shots you had during the round and dividing that by the amount of shots you took to complete the round. For example: thirty-six intended shots divided by seventy-two total shots equals a 50 percent intended shots statistic.

This type of intended versus unintended shot assessment is a clear judge of one's production level. As opposed to just getting up there with a hit-and-hope mentality, it can be used without bias or evaluation. Let's say there was a shot that required you to hit the ball twenty-five feet left of the hole. Well, some may say that you hit a poor shot, when the fact of the matter is that you intended to hit it there. This system validates the player for what he or she accomplished and opens the door to take responsibility and handle what needs to be handled. This system allows you to keep track of strengths and weaknesses so you can practice to improve your weaknesses and hit shots that you have positive proof are your strengths.

This five-step process eliminates mind-noise on the golf course and allows you, the golfer, to enjoy playing Atomic Golf.

KEEPING YOUR STATS

The table on the following page is designed for you to keep track of your intended versus unintended shots on the golf course. Let's utilize the table to demonstrate how to keep your stats on a hole.

The first four columns record what the physical conditions were when you played the shot:

1. Wind direction: from which direction is the wind coming? As it relates to the directions of a clock, twelve would be a head-on wind, three would be a cross wind from the right, and so on.

2. Strength of wind: is the wind strength gusting low, medium, or high?

3. Distance: how far are you from where you want the ball to go?

4. Lie: where is the ball laying? On the tee? In the rough?

The next three columns keep track of the type of shot you played:

5. Club: which club you chose for the shot.

6. Swing type: was the shot hit with a wood? Was it an iron shot?

7. Form: did the shot you hit require any special height or curvature? Or was it a standard shot?

The final column is your end result:

8. Intended or unintended column: place a check mark in this box if the ball ends up where you intended, or an X if it does not.

CHART KEY (See chart below for where items are entered onto scorecard)

1—<u>Wind</u> column 1–12

2—<u>Strength</u> of the shot—L/M/H

3—<u>Distance</u> in yards

4—<u>Lie</u>: the location of the ball

5—<u>Club</u> number (wood or iron)

6—<u>Swing Type</u> used

7—<u>Form</u> used

see codes below for items 1–7

8—Intended or Unintended: ✔ for intended, ✘ for unintended

9—Player's first putt: ✔ for make, ✘ for miss

10—Player's second putt (if necessary): ✔ for make, ✘ for miss

11—Player's third putt (if necessary): ✔ for make, ✘ for miss

12—Total number of putts on the green

13—Score on the hole

14—Line for the 2nd shot: repeat scoring items for numbers 1–7, non putt

15—Line for the 3rd shot: repeat scoring items for numbers 1–7, non putt

16—Line for the 4th shot: repeat scoring items for numbers 1–7, non putt

1 WIND	2 STRENGTH	3 DISTANCE	4 LIE	5 CLUB	6 SWING TYPE	7 FORM
Time Clock	L=Low	In Yards	T=Tee	Number	I=Ironshot	S=Standard
	M=Med		G=Ground	1-9,G,W,S,L	W=Woodshot	K=Knockdown
1–12	H=High		R=Rough		C=Chipshot	F=Fade
			B=Bunker		P=Pitchshot	D=Draw
			P=Hardpan		L=Lobshot	H=Hard
			U=Buried		X=Cut lobshot	

Where to enter above items on Scorecard

1ST HOLE	WIND	STRENGTH	DISTANCE	LIE	CLUB	SWING TYPE	FORM	INTENDED
	1	2	3	4	5	6	7	8
9 | 10 | 11	14							
12 | Putts	15							
13 | Score	16							

Sample Scorecard completed for 1st Hole

1ST HOLE	12	M	270	T	1	W	S	✔
✘ | ✔ |	12	M	150	G	8	I	S	✔
2 | Putts								
4 | Score								

	WIND	STRENGTH	DISTANCE	LIE	CLUB	SWING TYPE	FORM	INTENDED
1ST HOLE								
Putts								
Score								
2ND HOLE								
Putts								
Score								
3RD HOLE								
Putts								
Score								
4TH HOLE								
Putts								
Score								
5TH HOLE								
Putts								
Score								
6TH HOLE								
Putts								
Score								
7TH HOLE								
Putts								
Score								
8TH HOLE								
Putts								
Score								
9TH HOLE								
Putts								
Score								
TOTAL SCORE								

	WIND	STRENGTH	DISTANCE	LIE	CLUB	SWING TYPE	FORM	INTENDED
10TH HOLE								
Putts								
Score								
11TH HOLE								
Putts								
Score								
12TH HOLE								
Putts								
Score								
13TH HOLE								
Putts								
Score								
14TH HOLE								
Putts								
Score								
15TH HOLE								
Putts								
Score								
16TH HOLE								
Putts								
Score								
17TH HOLE								
Putts								
Score								
18TH HOLE								
Putts								
Score								
TOTAL SCORE								

Let's play the first hole. The wind is coming from straight-on twelve o'clock at medium strength. I want to hit it 270 yards off the tee with my driver with a standard swing. I hit it right where I wanted to, so I check off intended.

I get to the ball and the wind has not changed, it is still in my face from twelve o'clock at a medium strength. I intend to hit the ball 150 yards from off the ground (fairway) with an eight-iron, utilizing a standard swing. I hit it, and it ends up on the green. Again, I check off intended.

I miss my first putt, and make the second, noting that on the left side of the sheet with an X and a check mark. The next line records the total number of putts followed by the score for the hole.

At the end of the round, simply tally up the check marks, divide that number up by your total shots played, and you will have an intended stat for the day.

This form of statistical analysis allows a golfer to approach and achieve mastery in golf—a subject often discussed in golf as being unattainable. Well, with traditional golf, it is unattainable, but with Atomic Golf, it is quite real.

REDEFINING PERFECTION

Ben Hogan told reporters at the 1978 Masters Tournament that he had a dream of near perfection by having seventeen hole-in-ones and lipping out on the eighteenth. Perfection, some have stated, is shooting fifty-nine or better. This sort of arbitrary labeling of perfection is the reason the answer is left open to interpretation and debate.

In Atomic Golf, perfection is no less than creating 100 percent of your intended shots in the physical universe. The ability to duplicate your performance time and time again without strain or effort is a byproduct of mastery.

Before those definitions, David Duval's round of fifty-nine shot back in January 1999 on the PGA Tour would seem to be untouchable, yet the breakdown of intended shots versus unintended shots that day was approximately 83 percent. This is calculated by the result of his shots that day—he hit forty-nine out of fifty-nine shots to where he wanted them. Obviously, I can't speak on his behalf, but I'm sure he didn't intend to miss a putt that day nor did he miss a green intentionally.

This statistic highlights two things: 1) that there's actually 17 percent more to improve on a fifty-nine, and 2) shooting near par can often be done with 55 to 65 percent of intended shots going as you plan.

By keeping stats of your intended percentages, you can have a very real target to work on, and by using the information in this book, you strive toward reaching and surpassing that goal

THE ATOMIC GOLFER

Atomic Golf is creating a paradigm shift in the golf world. Its basic principles are grounded in truths that transcend the game of golf. The principles state that if a person has a clear mind and a fit body, then with the proper education in a given discipline (in this case, golf), the person has all the tools for becoming a champion.

As you now know, the Atomic Golf System challenges the way golf is instructed and played. It compresses the time, matter, energy, and space that it would normally take for a person to pick up this game and propels them years ahead without the detours or dead ends found with traditional instruction. You will be a powerful golfer in a shorter period of time.

The final product of Atomic Golf is a champion golfer, one who dominates the field of play and sends their opponents reeling into apathy. It is a being who has integrity and who takes on full responsibility for all aspects of their game. One who has dedicated himself or herself toward achieving all the small goals that accumulate and result in the big goals. One who has a never-say-die attitude on the golf course, where there are no alternate intentions. It is having the ability to take a mental image you have of the outcome, transmit it out of your head and through your body, and demonstrate it through your golf swing 100 percent of the time. What *you* want to do is what *you* do on the course.

Atomic Golf can be demonstrated. It is not another pie-in-the-sky theory that you read and glance over. Now, having read this book, your objective is to roll up your sleeves, get your mind and body in shape, do the drills in the correct sequence, then go out and apply what you have learned on the golf course.

Your authors have gone to great lengths to perfect the accumulated set of data before you here. The information in this book is 100 percent true. When applied correctly, you will get the intended result. See for yourself how true this is.

Afterword

It has been a great honor to work with Steve Michalik as coauthor on this project. I take my position of being the medium for the golf information with great pride and responsibility, and therefore I find myself very fortunate to present this book in unison with Steve, joining the technology of golf with Steve's knowingness of the mind and body.

Over the years, golf has provided me with wonderful opportunities and experiences, every time I have played it. I have met people from all walks of life, from different parts of the world, and yet we all have a common bond—the language of golf. With so much confusion and false data surrounding golf, to be able to contribute back to this sport with a truth that will empower others to experience the array of emotions golf can deliver is a special gift all by itself. My desire for a society that does not suppress the truth, but rather supplies a workable roadmap with individual responsibility to those who are willing to earn it, is a goal that transcends golf.

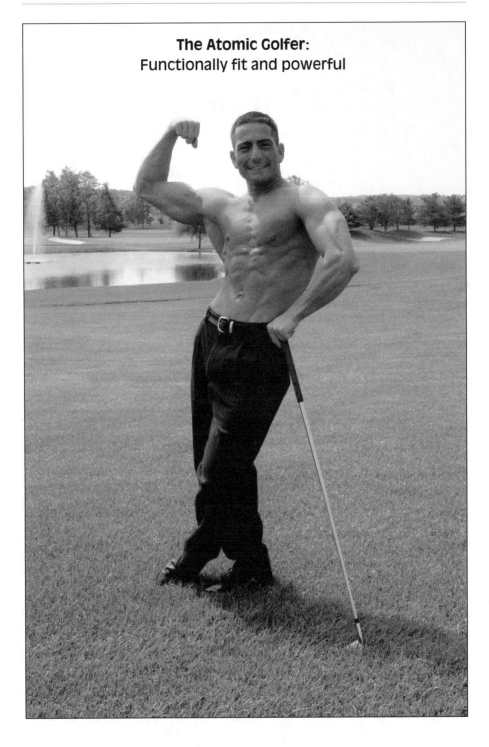

The Atomic Golfer:
Functionally fit and powerful

Testimonials

Perhaps one of the purest joys in life is to execute a perfectly hit golf shot. Interestingly, though, much can and cannot go into the execution of the "perfect" golf shot. Furthermore, what constitutes a perfect golf shot can also be debated. What I learned from the Atomic Golf System is what cannot be substituted for what really needs to happen: to make it all happen. There are an infinite number of ways a golf ball can fly once it is hit. However, only a good program can communicate to the reader what ingredients it takes to make a person understand and perfect a golf swing. I believe what makes such a program great is one that completely explains what it takes to produce a bad swing, in addition a good one, then armed with those tools the student can thereby carry on to produce a successful, fun, thrilling game of golf.

In *Atomic Golf*, Michael and Steve have pooled their vast compendium of knowledge on how the mind will create the golf swing and demonstrate it via the muscles of the body. Furthermore, this is why I elected *Atomic Golf* to be my source material in the game of golf. I would be remiss if I did not say that a swing is only part of the story. In "no-excuses" golf, one must understand the two other sides of the triangle, the mind and body. The combination of all three clearly gives me the confidence to execute any shot I need to produce. As a matter of fact, it has become a challenge and quite fun to call on these shots. *Atomic Golf* has reduced golf instruction to the simplest and most core components. Essentially, it is broken down into little pieces that are easily digested and remembered so I may reproduce them on my own. The confidence I now have in golf is second to none. No more first-tee jitters, no more hesitancy on club selection, in short . . . no more excuses. Through the teachings of proper equipment . . . yes, *Atomic Golf* covers all this too . . . to the strong and simple principles, I now can experience the golf I always dreamed about . . . big thanks, Michael and Steve.

James J. Burns
President and CEO, J. J. Burns & Company, LLC

Mike has done more research on the golf swing and has experimented with more trial-and-error attempts than anyone I've ever met. He knows what he is talking about, and it does work!

Brian Schuman
Multiple Winner, Golf Channel Amateur Golf Tour

As a chiropractor, I see an abundance of golf-related back injuries. *Atomic Golf* is the only bio-mechanically sound instruction available today that shows you how to hit a golf ball to prevent injuries. It creates a natural motion that is both powerful and stable and that rotates naturally around the spine. Combining this instruction with the muscle-building know-how from world champion Steve Michalik means you can ensure a lifetime of healthy and successful golf.

Durlan Castro, B.S., D.C., A.R.T.

The technology in *Atomic Golf* ushers in the new wave of golf instruction directed specifically at the twenty-first-century golfer. Utilizing functional muscles previously unheard of in the golf arena, the scientific principles found in *Atomic Golf* will revolutionize the sport and put golfers on the map as true athletes.

Scott Pounder
CEO, Nutrient Innovations
9 Handicap

Michael provides a unique perspective in the golf industry. Not only is he an accomplished player, but he is also an insightful instructor. Combine this with his successful approach to exercise and nutrition, and it makes him one of the foremost authorities in the field of golf fitness. This area will continue to expand and develop with his valuable input.

Allan Renz, Golf Instructor, Chelsea Piers Golf Academy
Teacher of the Year, Chelsea Piers 2003, 2004, 2005, 2006, 2007
Coach of the Year, Chelsea Piers 2005
Golf Range Magazine's Top 50 Golf Instructors in America in 2006

In a few short months, Steve converted me, a single mother who was once close to two hundred pounds and wearing a size twenty-two jean, into a natural bodybuilding champion—and all at the age of forty-one. Proving that anything is possible, Steve introduced me to Michael who asked if I had ever thought about playing golf competitively. I had never thought about being a bodybuilder, never mind a golfer, and within three short months, I broke 80 for the first time, and can't wait to play in state amateur events this summer.

Emanuela Silvagni
Professional Bodybuilder
WBBG Miss North America

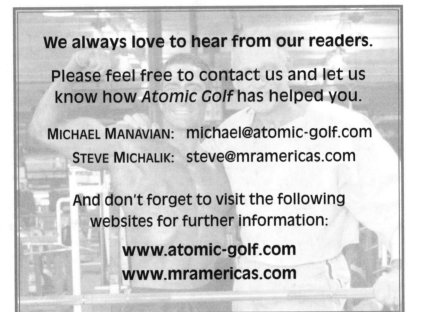

We always love to hear from our readers.

Please feel free to contact us and let us
know how *Atomic Golf* has helped you.

MICHAEL MANAVIAN: michael@atomic-golf.com

STEVE MICHALIK: steve@mramericas.com

And don't forget to visit the following
websites for further information:

www.atomic-golf.com

www.mramericas.com

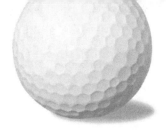

Resources

Clubfitters

Below is a worldwide listing of clubfitters by country and state. Be aware that addresses and telephone numbers are subject to change.

UNITED STATES

Alabama

Pro Golf Discount-Gulf Shores
3757 Gulf Shores Parkway, Gulf Shores, AL; (251) 968-8560

Alaska

Full Swing Golf of Alaska, 9360 Old Seward Highway, Anchorage, AK; (907) 344-4653

Arizona

Arizona Golf Exchange, 4877 E. Speedway Blvd., Tucson, AZ; (520) 325-8526

Eagle Flight Golf, 9821 W. Avenida Del Sol, Peoria, AZ 85383; (623) 581-5959

Golf Etc.-Chandler, 975 East Riggs Rd., Suite 9, Chandler, AZ; (480) 895-1992

Golf Etc.-Gilbert, 67 S. Higley Rd., Suite 108, Gilbert, AZ; (480) 497-4653

California

Bay Golf, 751 B. Camino Plaza, San Bruno, CA; (650) 588-9818

D.K. Golf Studio, 3732 West 6th St., Los Angeles, CA; (213) 388-0222

Faldo Golf Institute-Palm Desert, 9002 Shadow Ridge Rd., Palm Desert, CA; (760) 674-2737

Gold Country Golf, 11440 Sunrise Gold Circle, Suite 1, Rancho Cordova, CA; (916) 631-7025

Golf Coast Equipment & Supply, 1995 Ritchey St., Santa Ana, CA; (714) 259-7812

Golf Etc.-Corona, 2225 Eagle Glen Parkway #101, Corona, CA; (951) 310-1812

Golf Etc.-Fairfield, 104-A Commerce St., Fairfield, CA; (707) 864-6800

Golf Etc.-La Quinta, 79-305 Highway 111, Suite 5, La Quinta, CA; (760) 771-4488

Golf Excellence International, 11947 E. Florence #4, Santa Fe Springs, CA; (562) 879-5474

Golf Tech-CA, 659 S. Bernardo Ave., Sunnyvale, CA; (408) 732-8324

Joe McGowen Clubfitting-PGA West, 56-150 PGA Blvd., La Quinta, CA; (760) 564-3965

Joe's Custom Club & Repair, 75 Doray Dr., Pleasant Hill, CA; (925) 685-2524

K and J Golf, 5759-C Winfield Blvd., San Jose, CA; (408) 578-4100

Kepler's Golf, 2325 Boulevard Circle, Walnut Creek, CA; (925) 932-8179

King of Clubs Golf-CA, 9074 Elk Grove Blvd., Suite 5, Elk Grove, CA; (916) 685-3026

KZG Fitting & Training Center, 5125 Lankershim Blvd., North Hollywood, CA; (213)/(818) 762-3495

Lake Redding Golf Pro Shop, 1795 Benton Dr., Redding, CA; (530) 243-8527

Max 5 Sports, 18216 S. Western Ave., Gardena, CA; (310) 523-9058

Max Fit Golf, 401 S. Vermont Ave., Suite 14, Los Angeles, CA; (213) 252-0078

Menifee Lakes C.C., 29875 Menifee Lakes Dr., Menifee, CA; (951) 672-3090

Ocean Meadows Golf Course, 6925 Whittier Dr., Goleta, CA; (805) 957-9907

Pro Golf Discount-Simi Valley, 1472 E. Los Angeles Ave., Simi Valley, CA; (805) 520-9801

Springer Golf Productions, 647 Camino de Los Mares #108-258, San Clemente, CA; (949) 388-5163

TourTech, 279 S. Dillon Ave., Unit 1, Campbell, CA; (408) 871-8275

Colorado

John's Custom Clubs, 5750 S. Lemay, Fort Collins, CO; (970) 227-5044

Connecticut

Cote Golf Instruction LLC, Stamford Marriott Hotel, Stamford, CT; (203) 980-3423

East Windsor Golf & Practice Center, 12 S. Main St., East Windsor, CT; (860) 623-9422

Golf Etc.-New Haven, 163 Universal Dr., N., North Haven, CT; (203) 234-9086

Golf Training Center-CT, 145 Main St., Norwalk, CT; (203) 847-8008

Greenwich Golf Studio, 222 Mill St., Greenwich, CT; (203) 532-4810

Simsbury Farms G.C., 100 Old Farms Rd., W. Simsbury, CT; (860) 658-6246

Delaware

Club Craft Custom Golf, 3656 Silverside Rd., Wilmington, DE; (302) 479-0844

Florida

Club Foremations, 4456 S.E. Federal Way, Stuart, FL; (772) 463-1167

Custom Golf Products-Davenport, 45685 U.S. Hwy. 27, Davenport, FL; (863) 419-4653

The Fitting Center at Tiburon Golf Club, 2620 Tiburon Dr., Naples, FL; (239) 280-6366

Golf Ball Warehouse, 24181 S. Tamiami Trail, Bonita Springs, FL; (239) 948-9840

Golf Etc.-Lake Mary, 7025 C.R. 46A, Unit 1021, Heathrow, FL; (407) 833-4653

Golf Guys of Naples, 778 9th St., North, Naples, FL; (239) 793-2000

The Golf Learning Center, 6340 Techster
Blvd., Suite 2, Ft. Myers, FL;
(239) 280-6366

Golf Provisions, 7500 Ulmerton Rd.,
Unit 28, Largo, FL; (727) 536-8117

Lauden Golf-Ponte Vedra, 330 A1A N.,
Ponte Vedra, FL; (904) 543-1433

Lauden Golf-St. Augustine, 10950 U.S. 1
North, St. Augustine, FL;
(904) 429-0005

Mid-Florida Golf, 27615 U.S. Highway 27,
Suite 101, Leesburg, FL; (352) 315-8777

The Mitchell Tour Studio, 16301 Phil
Ritson Way, Winter Garden, FL;
(407) 905-2246

Mobile Golf Technology, 13177 42nd Rd.,
N., West Palm Beach, FL; (561) 714-5048

Palm Beach Golf Center, 3698 N. Federal
Hwy, Boca Raton, FL; (561) 395-1305

Shanes Golf Shop (aka Swing-Line Golf),
6220 Taylor Rd., Suite 104, Naples, FL;
(239) 594-1837

St. Lucie Golf Range, 6201 S. U.S.
Highway 1, Port St. Lucie, FL; (
772) 466-9968

Tee 2 Green-Delray Beach, 5859 W.
Atlantic Ave., Suite 89A, Delray
Beach, FL; (561) 638-2800

Tee 2 Green-Tamarac, 7148 N. University
Dr., Tamarac, FL; (954) 720-7780

World of Golf, 4500 Tamiami Trail N.,
Naples, FL; (239) 263-4999

Georgia

Golf Etc.-Acworth, 3450 Cobb Parkway
NW, Acworth, GA; (770) 975-3905

Golf Etc.-Mall of Georgia, 3276 Buford
Dr., Suite 108, Buford, GA;
(678) 714-5580

Golf Etc.-Pooler, 125 Foxfield Way, Suite
106, Pooler, GA; (912) 748-7200

Lake Oconee Golf Company, 601 Oak St.,
Eatonton, GA; (706) 484-0070

Malachi Custom Clubs & Repair,
1465 Dahlonega St., Cumming, GA;
(770) 889-9161

Shortgrass Golf, 3890 Floyd Rd., Austell,
GA; (678) 556-0705

Hawaii

Golf Stix-HI, 98-027 Hekaha St., Suite 27
Aiea, HI; (808) 487-1217

Illinois

Bloomington Indoor Golf, 11 Finance Dr.,
Suite 11, Bloomington, IL;
(309) 662-6439

Budget Golf-Joliet, 1508 Essington,
Suite 6, Joliet, IL; (815) 729-4653

The Club Shop-IL, 300 N. Greenbay Rd.,
Lake Forest, IL; (847) 234-8225

EJL Custom Golf Clubs, Inc., 825 75th St.,
Willowbrook, IL; (630) 654-8887

Golf Etc.-Shorewood, 217 N. Vertin Blvd.,
Shorewood, IL; (815) 609-9503

Ironwood Golf & Practice Center, 2322
N. Conger Rd., Pecatonica, IL;
(815) 239-2232

Pro Golf Discount-Crystal Lake, 6330
Northwest Highway, Crystal Lake, IL;
(815) 477-0000

Indiana

Custom Golf of New Haven, 10433
E. Paulding Rd., New Haven, IN;
(260) 749-5420

Fairway Custom Golf-Fishers, 12500
Brooks School Rd., Fishers, IN;
(317) 842-0017

Fairway Custom Golf-Greenwood,
681 S. Sheek Ave., Greenwood, IN;
(317) 859-1459

Fairway Custom Golf-Terre Haute,
1641 South 25th St., Terre Haute, IN;
(812) 478-3333

Golden Eagle Golf-IN, 8404 Brookville
Rd., Indianapolis IN; (317) 351-1263

Indy Custom Golf, 9830 Michigan Rd.,
Carmel, IN; (317) 228-0100

Speedway Custom Golf, 10117 E. U.S.
136, Indianapolis, IN; (317) 293-4200

Iowa

Golf Etc.-Ankeny, 1802 E. Delaware Ave.,
Suite 110C, Ankeny, IA; (515) 964-2025

Golf Etc.-Cherokee, 206 W. Main St.,
Cherokee, IA; (712) 255-2129

Kansas

Golf MD, 11505 S. Strang Line Rd.,
Suite A, Olathe, KS; (913) 663-5050

Louisiana

Academy Club Service at Money Hill,
100 Country Club Dr., Abita Springs,
LA; (985) 809-7170

Maryland

Adro's Custom Golf, 12111 Nebel St.,
Rockville, MD; (301) 570-9010

Golf Etc.-Annapolis, 302 Harry S. Truman
Parkway, Suite J, Annapolis, MD;
(410) 897-9500

Massachusetts

Fit to a Tee Custom Golf-MA, 928 D Route
28, S. Yarmouth, MA; (508) 398-4653

Profitters Golf, 167 Elm St., Agawam, MA;
(413) 789-9642

Pro Golf Discount-Shrewsbury, 1000
Boston Turnpike, Shrewsbury, MA;
(508) 842-0142

Michigan

Dale's Golf Shop, 6104 Angling Rd.,
Portage, MI; (269) 327-2155

Indian Hills Golf Course, 4887 Nakoma,
Okemos, MI; (517) 349-1010

Precision Golf-MI, 9975 E. Grand River,
Brighton, MI; (810) 225-4653

Minnesota

Golf Club Hospital, 4308 Bryant Ave., S.,
Minneapolis, MN; (612) 825-5389

Mississippi

Tee to Green Golf Custom Clubfitting,
10340 B D'Iberville Blvd., Diberville,
MS; (228) 396-4416

Missouri

Kelly's Golf Ltd., 7823 Olive Blvd.,
St. Louis, MO; (314) 725-4663

Montana

Mitchell Golf, 3007 Montana Ave.,
Billings, MT; (406) 245-8691

Nebraska

Classic Golf, 4617 Dodge St., Omaha, NE;
(402) 554-0202

Nevada

Golf Nut, 4275 N. Rancho Dr., Suite 155,
Las Vegas, NV; (702) 658-7787

Pro Golf Discount-Las Vegas, 510
Mark St., Ste 100, Henderson, NV;
(702) 433-9911

New Hampshire

Collins Kustom Club Fitting Center,
762 E. Industrial Park Dr., Suite 5,
Manchester, NH; (603) 623-7876

New Jersey

Club Doc, 1251 Jumping Brook Rd.,
Neptune, NJ; (732) 668-5210

Enterprise Golf & Sportswear, Inc.,
600 Secaucus Rd., Secaucus, NJ;
(201) 348-6544

Hamilton Golf Center, 5 Municipal Dr.,
Hamilton, NJ; (609) 581-0045

Hoboken Golf, 125 Grand St., Hoboken,
NJ; (201) 876-9666

Jack of Club/Hyatt Hills, 1300 Raritan
Rd., Clark, NJ; (732) 669-9265

Johnson's Golf Clubs, 1770 Rt. 34, North
Wall, NJ; (732) 681-1842

Perfect Swing, 3011 Route 37 E., Toms
River, NJ; (732) 929-4229

New Mexico

Dave's Golf Mart, 4200 Wyoming N.E.,
Albuquerque, NM; (505) 296-5866

New York

Gallagher Golf Direct, 1084 Morton Blvd.,
Kingston, NY; (845) 336-9341

Golfer's Edge, 2600 Baird Rd., Penfield,
NY; (585) 383-9280

Greater Golf Training Center, 225
Harrison Ave., Endwell, NY;
(607) 484-0147

Peak Performance Golf Training, 1
Pinerobin North, Greensfield Center,
NY; (518) 301-0791

Precision Golf Center, 651 Hayts Rd.,
Ithaca, NY; (607) 277-6353

Pro Golf Discount-Nanuet, 211-B West
Route 59, Nanuet, NY; (845) 624-2304

North Carolina

Arboretum Golf, 8020 Providence Rd.,
Charlotte, NC; (704) 542-5511

Golf Etc.-Wake Forest, 11829 Retail Dr.,
Wake Forest, NC; (919) 556-6411

The Golf Academy, 750 Auburn-
Knightdale, Raleigh, NC;
(919) 661-7100

The Golf Shop-Salisbury, 1953 Jake
Alexander Blvd., Salisbury, NC;
(704) 633-0333

J & S Custom Clubs, 3487 Lackey St.,
Lumberton, NC; (910) 739-7080

Kelly's Custom Golf, 1721 Battle Ground
Ave., Greensboro, NC; (336) 272-8572

Methodist University Golf Shop,
5400 Ramsey Street, Player Building,
Fayetteville, NC; (910) 630-7684

Pierson Drew Golf Ltd., 111 Summer
Haven Ave., Wilmington, NC;
(910) 256-4912

Randy's Golf Center and Range,
1706 Hanford Rd., Graham, NC;
(336) 570-3996

Special-Tee Custom Golf, 1620 E. Chester
Dr., Suite 103, High Point, NC;
(336) 889-0333

Steve's Golf Shop, 2648 Andrews Circle,
Lenoir, NC; (828) 726-0922

Ohio

Akron Golf Clubs, 396 E. Tallmadge Ave.,
Akron, OH; (330) 253-8000

Golf Stix-OH, 11772 Springfield Pike,
Cincinnati, OH; (513) 671-3033

McGolf, 14572 US 23 Suite D, Waverly,
OH; (740) 941-4653

Mulligan Golf, 1011 F. State Route 28, Milford, OH; (513) 831-8633

Murphy's Golf Repair, 770 N Main St., Akron, OH; (330) 253-9498

Ohio Valley Golf Center, 15415 State, Rt. 170, Calcutta, OH; (330) 386-6226

Rollandia Golf Center, 4990 Wilmington Pike, Dayton, OH; (937) 434-4911

Woods N Irons Driving Range, 3271 County Road M50, Edon, OH; (419) 272-3021

Oklahoma

Aberdeen Golf Company, 8821 S. Santa Fe Ave., Oklahoma City, OK; (405) 636-1666

Mason-Earle Golf & Gear, 205 Mimosa Lane, Tahlequah, OK; (918) 453-1117

Oregon

Club Crafters, 1020 Green Acres Rd., Suite 2, Eugene, OR; (541) 343-2222

North Woods Golf Company, 7410 S.W. Macadam Ave., Portland, OR; (503) 245-1910

Pennsylvania

84 Golf Center, 16 Golf Center Drive, Eighty Four, PA; (724) 229-4002

Clubmakers Shop, 1457 Stefko Blvd., Bethlehem, PA; (610) 865-9192

Dick Moyer Custom Golf at Mayapple, 194 Richwine Rd., Suite 2, Shermans Dale, PA; (717) 258-1910

Gigi Golf, 866 Concord Rd., Concordville, PA; (610) 558-4653

Golf Augusta–Oakmont, 607 B Allegheny Ave., Oakmont, PA; (412) 828-1580

Golf Etc.–Montgomeryville, 741 Bethlehem Pike, Montgomeryville, PA; (215) 361-2582

Golf Shop at Mad Golfer Driving Range, 114 Street Rd., Southampton, PA; (215) 357-1622

Rhode Island

Spargo Golf, 1 Keyes Way, West Warwick, RI; (401) 828-2857

South Carolina

Accelerized Golf of Lake Wylie, 5241 Charlotte Highway, Clover, SC; (803) 831-1101

Championship Golf, 1800 Business, 17, South Myrtle Beach, SC; (843) 215-0433

The Club Maker–SC, 10 B Johnson Way, Bluffton, SC; (843) 757-7636

Cobb's Gold Tee Golf Shop, 1731 Sandifer Blvd., Seneca, SC; (864) 888-8882

Dr. Golf-Pawley's Island, 10080 Ocean Highway, Suite 8, Pawley's Island, SC; (843) 237-3362

Tennessee

Golf and Tennis Express, 626 Simmons Rd., Knoxville, TN; (865) 966-3774

Greg Pickett Golf, Inc., 7849 Winchester Rd., Suite 102B, Memphis, TN; (901) 757-1112

Sweet Stix Golf, 1395-H Volunteer, Bristol, TN; (423) 968-4885

Texas

Custom Clubs By Larry Gibson, 11875 W. Little York, Suite 206 Houston, TX; (832) 467-9668

Golf By George, 1012 B Dallas Dr., Denton, TX; (940) 891-2633

Golf Etc.—Weatherford, 2124 Tin Top Rd., Suite 100, Weatherford, TX; (817) 613-1122

O'Brien's Golf, 23802 Highway 59, North Kingwood, TX; (281) 359-2627

Saturn Golf, 5610 Frankford Ave., Lubbock, TX; (806) 785-5363

Vermont

J.P. Larkin Golf Course, 130 Brookmeade Circle, White River Junction, VT; (802) 674-6491

Virginia

Affordable Golf at Owl's Creek Golf Center, 411 S. Birdneck Rd., Virginia Beach, VA; (757) 425-4653

Dynamic Golf Studio, 5251-47 John Tyler Highway, Williamsburg, VA; (757) 253-0589

Flagstick Custom Golf, 9936 Midlothian Turnpike, Richmond, VA; (804) 327-1600

Hodson Golf, 1405 East Look Lane Powhatan, VA; (804) 475-6311

Jim's Golf Shop at Sunnybrook, 8535 Sudley Rd., Manassas, VA; (703) 369-0070

NOVA Golf & Tennis, 14415 Potomac Mills Rd., Woodbridge, VA; (703) 494-6020

Pro Am Golf Company, 1409 Oriana Rd., Suite A, Yorktown, VA; (757) 890-9312

Spring Hill Golf, 16500 Midlothian, Midlothian, VA; (804) 794-7193

Total Performance Golf, 2626 West Main, Waynesboro, VA; (540) 949-8331

Washington

Golf Etc.-Vancouver, 6700 NE 162nd Ave. Suite 401, Vancouver, WA; (360) 944-8808

Vons Golf & Putter Studio, 2811 B NE 55th St., Seattle, WA; (206) 524-6716

Wisconsin

Gastraus Golf Center/Driving Range, 1300 East Rawson Ave., Oak Creek, WI; (414) 571-7002

Marshfield C.C., 11426 Wren Rd., Marshfield, WI; (715) 384-4409

Pro Shop at Verona Meadows, 2905 Shady Oak Lane, Verona, WI; (608) 845-3777

Wyoming

Golf Etc.-Cheyenne, 1740 A Dell Range Blvd., Cheyenne, WY; (307) 632-8051

CANADA

Al's Clubhouse, 6732 Cedar Acres Dr., Greely, Ontario; (613) 860-4653

Alberta Golf Works, 4699 61st St., Suite 5, Red Deer, AB; (403) 346-4653

Analyst Golf Shop, 9550 Bearspaw Dam Rd. NW, Calgary, AB; (403) 208-2206

Artisan Golf Co., 215 Terrace Mathews Crescent, Suite 3, Ottawa, Ontario; (613) 592-0524

Bluffs Golf Club, 35593 Lake Line Rd., Port Stanley, Ontario; (519) 782-7447

Camber Golf Equipment, 201 Enterprise Way, Kelowna, British Columbia; (250) 860-7772

Dog Leg Left Golf Services, 2401 Cliffe Ave., Suite 12, Courtenay, British Columbia; (250) 703-0440

ESP Fitting System, 16083 Hurontario, Caledon, Ontario; (800) 642-2212

Fore The Golfer, 134 Doncaster Ave. Unit #1, Thornhill, Ontario; (905) 709-2112

Golf Etc.-Niagara Falls, 3969 Montrose Rd., Unit 9, Niagara Falls, Ontario; (905) 374-4653

Golf Les Rivieres Inc., 6500 Blvd. Des Forges, Trois-Rivieres, PQ; (819) 378-7871

Golf Link-MB 855 Henderson Highway, Winnipeg, MB; (204) 663-2106

Golf Price Canada, Ste-Adele Quebec; (450) 229-4879

Golf West-Canada, 4061 B Norwell Dr., Nanaimo, British Columbia; (250) 758-1919

Grand Lynx Golf Center, 4301 Regional Rd. 35, Chelmsford, Ontario; (705) 560-6673

Harvest Hills Golf Center, 999 Country Hills Blvd., Calgary, Alberta; (403) 255-4653

Jeffersports, 1622 Pemberton Ave., North Vancouver, British Columbia; (604) 983-9898

King Custom Golf, 1501 8th St., Suite #2, East Saskatoon, SK; (306) 373-1808

McMahon Golf, 7370 Woodbine Ave., Unit 23, Markham, Ontario; (905) 479-1796

Newtons Law Golf at Peace Arch Driving Range, 765 172nd St., Surrey, British Columbia; (604) 535-6492

Oakville Golf, 360 Dundas St., East Bldg. B, Unit 7, Oakville L6H 6Z9; (905) 825-5757

Paradise Golf-Canada, 213 W. Frederica, Thunder Bay; (807) 628-0668

Ron Brown Custom Golf Works, 27 Director Court, Woodbridge, Ontario; (416) 578-6035

Swing-Rite Golf & Fitness, 4870 Bank St., South Ottawa, Ontario; (613) 852-4688

Taurus Golf Ltd.-MB, 1127 Brae Crest Dr., Brandon, MB; (204) 728-6967

Tayler Quality Golf, 20 Hartzel Rd. Unit #10 St., Catherines, Ontario; (905) 688-4653

Ted and Dave Custom Golf, 7100 15th St. SE, Calgary, Alberta; (403) 640-0082

Village Green, 8525 Conc. #2, Stoney Point, Ontario; (519) 798-4401

INTERNATIONAL CLUBFITTERS

Australia

Advantage Custom Clubmakers, 136 Willoughby Rd. Crows Nest, Sydney 2065 NS; 61 02 9966 4244

Golf Club Innovations-Queensland, 1/1 Stockwell Place, Suite 1, Archerfield, Queensland; 61 07 3373 8988

Golf Workshop, 405 High St., Ashwood, Victoria; 61 03 9885 1544

New Age Golf Solutions Pty Ltd Shop, 7 Benowa Place, 83 Ashmore Rd., Bundall, Queensland; 61 07 5592 3388

Statesman Golf-c/o Melton Golf Range, 11-15 Ferris Rd. Melton, Victoria; 61 03 9743 9189

Austria

Golfschule Sterngartl, Schauerschlag 4 Oberneukirchen 4181; 43 43721221328

Barbados

Worme Proverbs, Friendship Terrace
Lodge, Hill St. Michaels; 246 424-2974

Belgium

Golfan, 177A Chaussee De Binche Mons
7000; 32 65340540

Czechoslovakia

Golf Gate k.s., Na Hrazi 27, Praha 8;
420 420323617323

Germany

JWP-Golf, Hinter dem Turm 29, 55286
Woerrstadt; 49 6732934475

Trust Golf Oberuttkau, 4c Haarbach;
49 8535-911012

Hong Kong

Central Golf Company Ltd., B27-28,
Basement Fl., Bank of America Tower,
Hong Kong; 852 98211724

Improve Your Game Ltd., G/F 56
Leighton Rd. Causeway Bay,
Wanchai, Hong Kong; 852 28948338

Ireland

Donegal GolfWorks, Springfield, Glebe
Letterkenny, County Donegal;
353 (0)872398333

Pro-Fit Golf-Dublin, Newpark Shopping
Center, Unit 6, Blackrock, Dublin;
353 12783334

Italy

Golf Tecnica, Via Procaccini 45, Milan;
39 338-7167262

Japan

Golf World Net, 3-10-15 Koyama,
Nishiku, Kobe; 078 922-1900

Korea

Pro Tour Golf, 499-1 Yubang-Dong,
Yongin-Si Kyung Ki Do, Korea;
82 313227557

Tayoon Golf, #F-19 Sigma II Officetel
Bundang City, Korea, S. Korea;
82 31-726-0020

Woods Golf Fitting Center, 202-202
L'Park, 10-1 bunji, Jeongja-dong
Bundang-gu, Seongnam Si,
S. Korea; 82 317151235

Malaysia

Aswan Custom Clubs & Repair, Seksyen
U8 Bukit Jelutong Selangor, Shah Alam
Mala; 60 012-9339339

Old Clubhouse, 63 Jalan Bangkung,
Bukit Bandaraya, Kuala Lumpur;
60 2095 7133

Netherlands, The

FATco Golfclubs op maat, Marisplantsoen
8, Nieuwegein; 31 30 6034421

Golfusion Rimburgerweg, 50 6445 BA,
Brunssum; 003 0031(0) 624511511

New Zealand

Golf House at Manukau, Manakau Golf
Club, 1/1 Great South Rd., Takanini,
Auckland; 64 09 2675314

Golf House at Middlemore Auckland
Golf Club, Hospital Rd., Otahuhu,
Auckland; 64 09 2763722

Golf House Ltd., 10 Kingdon St.,
Newmarket, Auckland; 64 95 291930

Norway

Andersens Golf i Nord, Bjrne Erlingsons
Gt St., Harstad; 47 9013-8884

Custom Golf-Norway, Snaroyavei
69, Snaroya, Norway; 47 9087-2659

Philippines

Custom Clubmakers Intl., 520 Shaw
Blvd., Cor Old Wack Wack Rd.
Mandaluyong City; 63 2-718-3151

Custom Clubmakers Intl., Makati Golf
Club, 7232 Malugay St., Makati City;
63 2-830-2222

St. Lucia

St. Lucia Golf & CC., Cap Estate Grosilet,
St. Lucia, St. Lucia; 758 450-8523

Singapore

Falcon Golf Technology, 154 West Coast
Rd., Ginza Plaza #01-132, Singapore
127371; 6563410700

My Golf Shop Pte Ltd., Unit 01-02 Bukit
Timah Plaza/1 Jalan Anak Bukit,
Singapore; 656 463-4334

Spain

Golfplanet, Calle Antoni Maura 63 07620,
Llucmajor-Mallorca; 34 636028543

Practigolf Riviera, Mirafiores Golf
Academy Ave., Esmeralda S,
N Riviera Del Sol; 34 95293981

Sweden

Akersberga Golf Course, Bransle Gard,
184 26 Akersberga Stockholm;
46 8 540 691 70

Bosjokloster Golfstore, Bosjokloster
GolfklubbHoor; 46 4132 5860

Flog & Birdie Sports of Stockholm,
Observatoriegatan 7, Stockholm;
46 85 454 0899

SwingFit, Snickarv, 9 15335 Jarna;
46(0)855150058

Switzerland

Pepe's Golf Clinic, Schoenenhofsrasse
17 CH - Frauenfeld; 41 527216762

Taiwan

King Yang Company, 277 Tunglin West
Rd., Linyuan Shiang, Kaohsiung;
886 7 6429985

Thailand

Buyshaftdot.com, Ltd., 5/1316 Sasmakki
Rd., Pak Kret Nothaburi;
66 1-304-8989

Custom Clubmakers Company Ltd., 2/Fl
13/1-2 Selakam Rd,. PO Box 10, Hua
Hin Prachuabkirkhan; 66 3253-0119

GMT Clubmakers Deluxe, 44/447
Nawamin Rd. Klongkum, Bungkum,
Bangkok; 66 (0)2-947-8663

United Kingdom

Applied Golf Technology, 3 Main St.,
Ceres, Cupar Fife, Scotland;
44 1334828090

Club Masters–England, Dundry
Nurseries, Bamfurlong Lane,
Cheltenham, England; 44 1452-715007

Golfmark, Parley Golf Centre/Hurn, Nr.
Bournemouth, Dorset, England;
44 1202593106

Huntercomb Golf Shop at Huntercomb
Golf Club, Nuffield Henley on Thames,
England; 44 1491641241

Venezuela

Todogolf, C.A., Urbanizazion Chulavista
Calle Icabaru Resd, Sierra Nevada
PH2B; 58 212-2676882

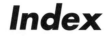

Index

About the Authors

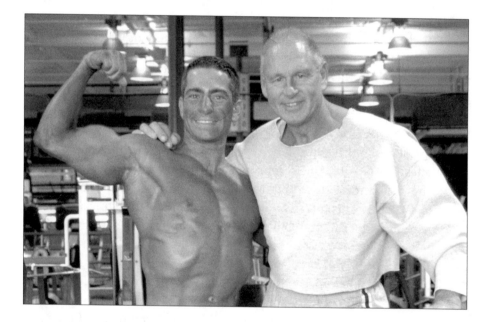

Steve Michalik, right, a triple-crown bodybuilding champion, whose titles include Mr. USA, Mr. America, and Mr. Universe, among twenty-two various others, began developing his Atomic Intensity System of training as a youth. Due to an abusive childhood, Michalik spent most of his time locked in a closet with nothing to occupy him but a stack of super-hero comic books. A scrawny kid with bad genes, a small bone structure, and low self-esteem, Michalik dreamed of becoming like his hero, Captain America, who was larger than life, and stood for courage, strength, integrity, and a love of country. Thus, was born Steve's quest for knowledge, truth, and the ultimate answers in the pursuit of how to build the ultimate physique.

Growing up, Michalik was fortunate enough to come in contact with people who could assist him in his quest. His family physician, Dr. Merkin, was the first to offer guidance, and was a great inspiration to Michalik. Dr. Merkin mentored Michalik, not only in the areas of anatomy and physiology, but also on the important roles of philosophy and spirituality in overcoming life barriers. Dr. Merkin's vast library introduced Michalik to the teachings of the Bible as well as the works of Darwin, Newton, Aristotle, Socrates, Plato, and Shakespeare, all of which he consumed voraciously. Michalik was determined to not only learn the mechanics of the mind and body, but also the "whys" behind their functions. Michalik was driven to search for truth, rather than accepting popularly promoted appearances. It was this drive that would set forth the basic law he would follow for the rest of his life: "agree to disagree." Unbeknownst to Michalik, at this early stage, it would be this point of view that would enable him to achieve championship status, and eventually, even save his life.

A further inspirational figure in Steve's journey was his Uncle John. Steve's uncle was a physicist who worked at Area 51, a parcel of U.S. military-controlled land in southern Nevada, apparently containing a secret aircraft testing facility. Uncle John was a treasure trove of information regarding time, space, energy, and matter. Michalik immediately realized the applicability of this information to muscle growth, and quickly assimilated these principles to bodybuilding. This revolutionary system of training would become what is now known today as Atomic Intensity, or, as coined by the *New York Times*, Atomic Fitness.

Steve's insatiable appetite for knowledge and truth compelled him to seek out many spiritual leaders and great minds of the world. While serving in the armed forces in Southeast Asia, Michalik would spend much of his off-duty hours in the mountains with Buddhist monks, learning all he could about their philosophy, and how they utilized the powers of the mind. The rest of his time was spent, against the direct command of superior officers, lifting cement-block barbells in the open fields. When told how dangerous this was, Michalik would simply explain that he couldn't be killed; after all, he had a destiny to fulfill. He was destined to become Mr. America.

Michalik fulfilled this destiny in his early twenties. After winning the titles of Mr. USA, Most Muscular Man in the USA, and various other competitions, Michalik achieved the extremely rare honor of being awarded the title of Mr. America his first time out. After proceeding to win the prestigious title of Mr. Universe in 1975 with his 250 pounds of perfectly symmetrical muscle, Michalik was primed to win Mr. Olympia and put an end to Schwarzenegger's reign. His escalating fame and popularity, prompted a network to offer him a spot hosting a science show, and he was filmed extensively for the movie "Pumping Iron." Steve's future seemed certain, when suddenly, tragedy struck. Failing to notice Steve's Mustang, the driver of a dump truck backed his vehicle over it, crushing the car and Steve's spine. Paralyzed from the waist down, doctors were convinced Michalik would never walk again. It was at this time that Steve's "mind over body" abilities would be put to the ultimate test.

Remaining true to his philosophy—agree to disagree—Michalik was determined to prove the doctors wrong. He would use the power of the mind to achieve the "impossible."

With the help of his eight-year-old brother, Paulie, Michalik embarked on a plan of rehabilitation. Each night, at the ungodly hour of 2 A.M., Michalik and Paulie would battle their way to the car. With Paulie hunkered below, working the gas and brakes, and Michalik at the wheel, the team of brothers made their way to a friend's gym in Amityville, New York. There, with Paulie's assistance, Michalik would drag himself from machine to machine, never giving in to self-doubt, or allowing for any consideration other than success.

The doctors predicted it would be at least ten years, if ever, before the nerves in Steve's legs began to come back to life. Michalik was thrilled then, when after only a few months, pain began developing in his lifeless limbs. Disagreeing with the increasingly excruciating pain, Michalik pushed harder, until he was leg pressing 800 pounds. A year later, in Florida, displaying 30-inch thighs and a 27-inch waist, Michalik shocked the audience when he appeared as the last contestant in a Grand-Prix show and was awarded a slot in the tour! Arnold Schwarzenegger, who was hosting the production, couldn't believe his eyes as he gasped, "It's Steve Michalik, the phantom bodybuilder." From that point on, Michalik would forever be known as "The Phantom."

Michalik's philosophy of mind over body, in combination with his principles of Atomic Fitness, enabled him to achieve tremendous success, and conquer enormous physical and mental barriers. His system of Atomic Intensity has proven its effectiveness time and again, both in his personal career, as well as the careers of other well-known champions. Some well-known names Michalik has had the privilege to work with include body-building champions Lou Ferrigno (The Hulk) and John DeFendis (Mr. America), author/bodybuilder Joyce Vedral, the Swiss Olympic Track Team, as well as baseball and football legends Darryl Strawberry and Lyle Alzado, to name a few.

Today, Michalik teaches the principles of Atomic Fitness, compressing time, space, and energy to increase matter, to a bevy of time-strapped full-time homemakers and corporate leaders. Michalik's clients are constantly amazed at their ability to transform their physiques in a fraction of the time they were previously investing. He is the author of *Atomic Fitness* (Basic Health, 2006), a comprehensive guide to the psychological and physiological aspects of this unique system of training.

Michalik has been written about in the *New York Times*, *Sports Illustrated*, *Newsday*, and numerous other newspapers and magazines. He has appeared on several dozen television programs, has been interviewed on radio talk shows, and has received honors and awards for his longstanding campaign against the use of steroids and his promotion of bodybuilding and fitness.

Michael Manavian, a graduate from the Professional Golf Management Program at Methodist College, is currently a personal golf coach to many around the country. Through the Internet he is able to keep in touch with his students via email and video conferencing in order to keep all of his clients playing to their peak. His impressive list of students includes PGA Tour players, U.S. Men's and Women's amateur qualifiers, New York City Amateur Champions, PGA Club professionals, and USGA state team members. A former playing member of the TearDrop Professional Golf Tour, he has competed in over 200 professional tournaments around the country. In 2004, he started Manavian Golf, a manufacturing company that designs and builds high-tech putters, which have been used by PGA Tour professionals.

Along with his golf schedule, in 2005 Manavian ventured into the sport of bodybuilding and won his class at the NPC Natural Northern USA, NPC Bev Francis' Atlantic States, and placed runner-up in the IFBB North American Championships, along with two best poser awards.

Manavian has published articles in *Golf Illustrated*, *The Met Golfer*, and several other magazines. He co-developed the Atomic Golf System in conjunction with co-author Steve Michalik. *Atomic Golf* is his first book.

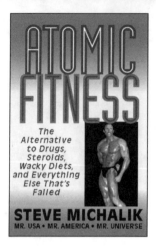
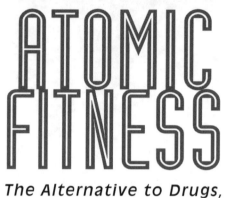